The Art of Baby Making

by Gerad Kite

Published by New Generation Publishing in 2013

Copyright © Gerad Kite 2013

First Edition

www.newgeneration-publishing.com

 New Generation **Publishing**

There is a crack in everything

– that's how the light gets in

- Leonard Cohen

Introduction

Our love of babies and instinctive need to procreate are the most powerful driving forces of humanity. The desire to see the next generation flourish is hardwired into our DNA and even those of us who, for whatever reason, do not have children, depend on and enjoy what the next generation brings. In recent years, troubled by falling fertility rates, we humans have started to dabble in the baby-making business as Western medicine has decided that infertility is a modern problem in need of a modern solution. Yet, when it comes to baby-making we really are amateurs; nature has been doing this job since the beginning of time.

The Art of Baby Making invites you to look at fertility and conception in a positive and transformational new light. Fertility rates in the West for both men and women are at an all time low and we are less in touch with nature than ever before. The book is about all people, and not just those who want to have children. The issues surrounding this epidemic of infertility are far bigger than you might think. They're a reflection of the general quality of life of prospective parents. As modern life provides our every material need and technology brings the world directly into our homes, our creativity and discovery of self is starting to be seriously compromised.

For over twenty years I've been working with both men and women in all kinds of relationships who have not been able to conceive and realise a child of their own. For many this journey is painful, frustrating and deeply saddening, but worst of all, it often gives people

6

a great sense of injustice, as though they've been shut out of a "normal" life through no apparent fault of their own. The hopelessness that many feel as each month and year rolls on is often rooted in a growing belief that they have somehow been excluded from the great plan of procreation. This touches a deep and dark part of us, and reminds us of the pain of feeling separate from others and different.

Everyone has a unique experience. I've worked with people who have damaged fallopian tubes or low sperm counts, and with people who struggled with long-term physical health problems that they thought were unrelated to their infertility. Often there's something emotional or psychological that is getting in the way.

"My husband and I had a vision of having kids and a family and we assumed it would happen the natural, easy way, and when it didn't it was a big shock. It was hard for me to get my head round it and work out what we could do next. It's hard on your relationship because you have to re-evaluate what it means for you." Joanne.

The UK alone has a "Fertility Industry" worth around £550,000,000 a year, with over 11,000,000 diagnosed infertile couples across Europe. Globally there are around 2,200 licensed medical clinics offering a variety of services such as in-vitro fertilisation (IVF), intra-cytoplasmic sperm injection (ICSI), egg donation, sperm donation and even treatments to suppress a woman's immune system in case it's attacking newly implanted embryos. You can take special fertility supplements made of high-dose vitamins or algae, or stock up with homeopathic remedies and follow a diet calculated to maximise your baby-making potential. There are travel companies offering "fertility retreats" where couples have massages and do yoga and qi gong.

Once a year at one of the largest exhibition halls in London, you can attend The Fertility Show where many of the clinics and practitioners specialising in fertility have stands and give out leaflets. You see bedraggled, dazzled looking couples wandering around with handfuls of leaflets offering competing packages of treatments and counselling and pampering. You can even have a fertility horoscope drawn up to calculate the right time to have sex and conceive.

Meanwhile the headlines bring new scare stories every day: "Sperm counts falling!", "Are women leaving it too late to have a baby?", "IVF babies born with fertility problems!", "Are you secretly infertile and don't know it?", "Infertility epidemic sweeps the Western world!". Friends suggest old wives tales; standing on your head after sex or eating kiwi fruit "because it's good for fertility", and your mum mutters that they didn't have these problems in her day and a colleague at work unhelpfully says she only has to look at her husband to get pregnant.

"The awful thing about infertility is you feel very unfeminine when everyone else is getting pregnant and you can't. It makes you feel like a complete failure as a woman. You feel very guilty that you're doing something bad and that's why it's not working. You think if only I'd had that vitamin or if I hadn't had that stressful phone conversation half an hour before the

treatment. You become paranoid about everything that you do." Elizabeth.

"It can be the hardest thing in the world when people turn round and say, 'Look at your daughter – she's so beautiful and you're so blessed to have her,' while they're surrounded by their three children, and you almost want to ask them how they'd react if one of their children were taken away from them. Secondary infertility is hard because you know what you're missing. These little beings are such cherubs and such incredible human beings. It can be difficult to realise that you won't do what you always thought you would, and have more, so you will literally do anything to change that". Valerie

In the middle of this onslaught of advice and advertising and recommendations and counter-recommendations it's hard to know how to stand back and calmly decide what you want to do when you are having difficulty conceiving, especially when your emotions are running high. What should be the simplest thing in the world has suddenly become a maze of options.

People with infertility issues often find themselves on a conveyer belt of treatment: first, when trying naturally fails, they are tested and diagnosed, then put on drugs to enhance ovulation. Then there's intrauterine insemination, to give nature another helping hand, and if and when that fails, IVF and then ICSI, when a single sperm is injected directly into a waiting egg in a Petri dish, and the resulting embryo returned to the mother for implantation.

If several cycles fail one can look into egg or sperm donation – an option complicated by a shortage of donors and difficulties with implantation – or begin, belatedly and in a demoralised state, the long path to adopting a child.

Over the years I've worked with a huge number of patients who have had children after reaching one stage or the next of this conveyor belt, and while I think there's nothing wrong with offering medical help to couples who have difficulty conceiving, sometimes this kind of intervention wasn't needed in the first place. The achievements of modern medicine can be little short of miraculous (and many of the people I see come for acupuncture while they go through a process like IVF or ICSI or the implantation of a donor egg), but I do believe that many of these clinics don't take into account the whole person, at great cost.

The majority have a very linear, logical approach, which deals only with the basic mechanics of introducing gamete to gamete and hoping that they "take" and it can leave the newly dubbed "patients" feeling dispirited and hollow. They've been sidelined as a couple, and they're "sick" or "faulty" and mysteriously "wrong" when they'd thought they felt well in themselves only a few months before.

In 2006 the Human Fertilisation and Embryology Authority reported that only 28.6 per cent of IVF cycles performed on women under the age of 35 ended in the birth of a baby. For older women, the success rate was still worse. There is a great deal of mystery around the low success rate of IVF, even when healthy embryos are created for implantation. It's understandable that we're so concerned about infertility being epidemic, and that medical treatment isn't a guaranteed solution.

Around twenty five per cent of all people who visit fertility clinics come away with an "unexplained infertility" diagnosis, and ten percent are told they are simply infertile. Every test has been run and no physical reason can be found for the couples' failure to conceive; the woman is ovulating, the man producing sperm, everything seems to be set up and ready to go, and yet there's no child.

It's a doctor's job to give a definitive answer to this conundrum, so unexplained infertility is an unsatisfactory diagnosis for them, leaving nothing to pinpoint and calibrate and finally "cure". To the patient it's a sword of Damocles. Nothing apparently is wrong with their bodies, but something is wrong with them and nobody can tell them what it is. There are plenty of suggestions; not enough salmon in your diet, too much salmon, shorts too tight, ovaries just need a boost. The search for a reason can be an endless parade of possibilities, and it feels like a tremendously personal diagnosis, leaving no one to blame but yourself.

It is also regularly reported that a large percentage of "older" women, those over the age of 35, go through fertility problems, but only a tiny percentage of those women have passed through the menopause, so there is no reason other than the controversial "ageing eggs" question as to why conception should be so difficult. We only know that despite great advances made in over-all health, fertility is not guaranteed as many couples discover, and natural selection works in its own mysterious way.

Let's face it, getting pregnant should be easy. People get pregnant without meaning to all the time. Two healthy human beings of childbearing years come together and have sex, and, given the right timing and conditions, the egg and the sperm meet and new life begins. Mother Nature makes the babies and does everything in her power to perform her art, unless something or someone gets in her way.

Maybe it's how we're living our lives, or what we are eating, or how we are feeling each day, maybe it's just bad luck, but from my experience it's normally something we can change – so we need to pay close attention if we want to be in the optimum state to work with nature and increase our chances of having a child.

Nature teaches us that a balanced state is a fertile state; and in this book I would like to share with you how "balance" can be the secret to successful conception, even when all else has failed. I will help you recognise if you are in balance, and if not, suggest ways to achieve it.

This word "balance" is loosely defined as a state of equilibrium and we are familiar with its usage in expressions like "work/life balance", "a balanced diet", "a balanced mind", and so on. However it is easy to oversee the subtlety of this natural phenomenon and forget that everything in life must be balanced in order to function well. For example, each day is balanced by night, winter is balanced by summer, men balance women, and one of the outcomes of this particular pairing is the creation of new life – a baby.

Unexplained Infertility

In my experience, the cause of "unexplained infertility" is rarely just a physical, medical condition but more often than not something emotional or even spiritual. In the Western world we've created a society that often undermines us as unique individuals and distances us from who we truly are. We struggle in a way that previous generations did not, and even though we live in a world of relative peace and prosperity where our chances should be better than ever, they are not. The more our lives become "spiritually" unbalanced this problem of infertility is unlikely to go away, and although advances in medical technology allow some couples to override the issue and conceive anyway, they may later find that they have yet to deal with that original problem manifesting itself as something else.

A lot of people react negatively when they hear the word "spiritual". They think you're talking about religious faith, or something mystical, but the meaning of "spirit" as understood in the philosophy that underpins Five-Element acupuncture and many other ancient healing traditions is something very different. In these systems of medicine, health and fertility are achieved by maintaining a balance of body, mind and spirit. "Body" is our actual physical form and "mind" is less tangible and more mysterious. Our "mind" creates our perceived reality through thought and feelings and constructs our life through experience and memories and is responsible for processing ideas. Everyone understands the "body" and "mind" of that equation, before shying away from the third. "Spirit" is our "being" or "self", intangible and beyond thought, form, time, and a sense of our own existence; "spirit" is the root and balancing point of everything.

If you and your partner are having trouble conceiving and there is no apparent medical cause then surely there must be something at play? To compare yourself with others who have conceived in what appears to be as a similar situation to your own is frankly pointless and disheartening. We are all different: our genetic history, our personal history, our friendships, our hopes and fears.

In this book I will explain how the balance of your body, mind and spirit is crucial to your fertility. Our very being on all levels is an environment that will give its best when all the elements of existence are present and in balance. Yes, some people are able to conceive despite having problems, but if you have had a verdict of "unexplained infertility" or there are other diagnoses that make conception harder for you, then you can increase your chances by taking a fresh look at yourself and do everything you can to be as well as is humanly possible. When we talk about making babies we are talking about a very natural process. When we tap into the abundance of nature, which celebrates itself by reproducing, we can be as well as humanly possible.

"Unexplained infertility" to my mind is nothing more than a label and not a state of being into which you've sunk, nor is it a chronic or intractable condition. This label however serves as an alarm bell that tells us something is wrong and more often than not the answers are there to be found - if only we knew where to look. This is what I want to talk about in this book. It's why this book is not your average fertility guide. It asks some big questions and brings up some big concepts.

There are many excellent guides to conception and conventional fertility treatments available which will give you a detailed account of what to expect when you embark on using one treatment or another, and which will help you make informed choices. What I hope to do in this book is to offer another perspective that can help you achieve a successful outcome and greatly improve your life as a whole. It takes a philosophical rather than a prescriptive approach and, hopefully, serves as a fertility enhancing experience in itself.

Many of the people I see need medical intervention to have children, and I have nothing against the use of these when there is a clear diagnosis that supports the chosen treatment. I just advocate a balanced perspective. Hormonal treatments can be physically and emotionally tough to endure, and you have to remain both optimistic and aware of the odds of success. I am concerned at times with the way that the mainstream fertility industry works, and particularly the way that many patients are encouraged to seek assisted fertility far too early to my mind, and how patients can be abruptly treated or dismissed by some clinics and consultants. In spite of these concerns, when appropriate, I have witnessed amazing results thanks to medical treatment.

My primary intention when working with

individuals either one on one or by sharing with you in this book, is to help awaken and discover the truth of who you really are. As you begin to recognise and break old habits, and dispel myths and unhelpful ideas that burden your mind, you will start to make choices that speak best to your true sense of self. This resulting level of personal awareness and clarity brings health on all levels. By being authentic, you will find a renewed sense of balance that will realign you with everything, which is a far better approach than trying to do it alone. There are no buttons that will simply switch fertility on or off. The relationship of the human body, mind and spirit are as complex as nature itself.

My job and the job of everyone in the fertility industry, be they a doctor, psychotherapist, acupuncturist or friend or family member, is to help move the person to a balanced place where the natural force of creation can dominate, resulting in a successful pregnancy. The energy that creates and sees life thrive is available to all of us equally. We simply need to provide the right conditions within ourselves to allow this life force to circulate and nourish throughout.

Every day in my work I see people improving in their physical and mental health, changing their lives for the better and often falling pregnant in spite of an earlier diagnosis of "unexplained infertility". However, I am not blind in my optimism; I'm a pragmatist too. It's not enough to simply turn up and receive this or that treatment. A certain focus, rigour and determination are needed to become a "healthy instrument" and the potential for a life-changing shift is there in you, whether it results in you having longed for children, or just living a better, happier life.

Case Studies

People come to professionals like me with many different problems and leave with many different solutions. Throughout this book I will use stories from people I have helped which I hope will show that infertility isn't a simple issue, but one that requires a holistic approach, which takes you, and many aspects of your life into account. Some will be brief accounts, and others more detailed case studies provided from the perspective of the people themselves. All of these stories reach a conclusion, but the outcomes are often surprising. They will guide you in how to overcome most obstacles and how to find your own path through the choices before you, and to emerge at the other end of your journey feeling more at peace and better in your own skin.

I will also use these stories to highlight how certain beliefs and ways of thinking can be counterproductive to your fertility; how to recognise these negative thought patterns in you, and how to make positive change. I will share the anecdotal evidence I have collected over many years that clearly helped the people who found success.

I will explain the Five-Element philosophy that underpins the acupuncture treatment that many of these people received. This explanation will show how the ancient wisdom contained in this system of medicine can be hugely beneficial to you, even without the insertion of a needle. While the philosophy behind the Five Elements may seem alien at first, I hope to demonstrate how it underlies even our western, twenty-first century lives.

A Holistic Approach

Jeanie and Nick Gordon had been together for seven years before they married in 2000, and twelve months later they began trying for a baby. Jeanie was 31 and Nick 34, and both of them had good jobs that they loved in London and had been able to buy their own flat. It seemed like the perfect set up for starting a family and everything had gone according to plan, but two years on there had been no positive pregnancy tests, and the couple felt surrounded by friends who were producing babies and even second babies without any problems.

Their GP referred them to a specialist who examined and tested both of them and found that Nick's sperm were not very active, and that Jeanie hadn't ovulated on her last cycle. A scan revealed that Jeanie had a large fibroid, which had twisted one of her Fallopian tubes back on itself. An operation to remove it worked, and after a month off work to recover, Jeanie felt refreshed and hopeful about the chances of becoming pregnant now that her physical problems had been cleared up. She carried on with her timetabled visits to the gym and with the vitamin supplements she'd been recommended, cutting back on alcohol just to be careful. Nick drank rather more and smoked a packet of cigarettes each day, but both the couples' GP and their consultant assured them that it would probably be stressful and therefore harmful for Nick, a committed smoker, to quit the habit.

Six months later, the couple had not conceived and Jeanie was under increasing stress. A friend who already had a child had just tested pregnant with twins. Although Jeanie had never experienced bad PMT, she now began to go through an enormous emotional and physical crash each month when her period began, and end up sobbing under her duvet or drinking too much and being so hung-over the next day that she had to phone in sick until her hormones had lapsed back to normal. Nick was hugely supportive all this time, but the couple was advised by their GP to move onto IVF. Jeanie had just moved jobs from a place where she'd had difficulties, and hoped that the change would remove some of the stress.

Jeanie started taking large doses of the hormone Clomid so that some of her eggs could be gathered and fertilised with Nick's sperm. The side effects of the hormones were grim – constant abdominal pain and mood swings – but the couple was determined to see it through. They were using ICSI, so only a few quality sperm would be needed once separated by the doctors in the laboratory and all Nick had to do was produce a sample. Although she felt under huge pressure, Jeanie reacted well to the treatment and produced a good quantity of eggs, most of which were frozen after fertilisation for future rounds of ICSI.

They were overjoyed when Jeanie tested pregnant after their first attempt. However, an early scan indicated problems with the foetus, and at eight and a half weeks Jeanie miscarried while staying at her sister's house. As her sister had just announced that she'd gotten pregnant after only three months of trying, Jeanie concealed what had happened from her, even driving herself to hospital with crippling stomach cramps. She later said that it felt like all her hope had gone with the pregnancy. Although her boss was understanding, going back to work was still difficult as the new job wasn't working out, she was being bullied by a colleague and waking up every night in panic.

Half a year later they tried a second round of ICSI, and this time when Jeanie conceived she carried on using hormone patches to help the pregnancy. Six weeks in, the scan showed that the foetus had been lost and Jeanie broke down in the car as they drove home. They had had enough. Jeanie was exhausted and exasperated at bearing the burden of the treatments, and was beginning to feel that her own body had let her down. They both knew that something had to change.

Jeanie had been looking at fertility treatments in acupuncture, reflexology and Chinese herbs. When a friend recommended our clinic, she decided to book an appointment for herself and Nick. At this stage, they hoped that acupuncture would help support further ICSI procedures and give the embryo a better chance of implanting. I saw the couple jointly for an initial consultation, and then separately for their actual treatment. Jeanie describes her experiences:

"Some of the tips given to us seemed very practical and straightforward, things like drinking more water and less coffee, but Gerad also tackled Nick on the question of his health and the link with his low sperm motility. Nick never ate breakfast or lunch, in fact he often didn't eat till 10 o'clock at night, and he was dreadful at getting out of bed in the morning. At the

weekends he'd sleep in till two in the afternoon. Gerad's advice to him was to eat a bacon sandwich for breakfast every morning, which of course Nick thought was fantastic. I thought it was fantastic too as over the weeks, I saw his energy levels changing. He was less sluggish in the mornings, and got up earlier at weekends.

To me it was a huge relief that he wasn't let off the hook any more. With the fertility treatments we'd had earlier, all he'd had to do was provide a couple of samples, but now for the first time it really felt like we were in it together. I poured my heart out, and it was so nice to sit down with somebody and let off steam that I even ended up with a parking ticket and didn't mind. The consultants we'd seen at the hospital had been great, but there was just something different about this – you didn't feel like you were out in the cold any more. It also felt like it was the whole of me that was being treated, and not just the baby making bits.

During the first treatment I remember having needles put in points down my back and left in for a while, and it felt like someone was pouring a jug of cold water over my back. It was a really weird sensation. Afterwards I felt positively trippy. It was like being on holiday, when you've forgotten to worry about everything and things look different; instead of saying "Oh God, look at the traffic", you're all "Oh! Cars! How lovely!" I asked him to tone it down a bit the next time! I began to get the sense that it would all work out ok.

After a couple of sessions we went away on holiday

and that was when I decided to give up work, and I don't think I'd have had the courage to walk out if it hadn't been for the acupuncture. I was a bit disappointed that I didn't turn out to be pregnant on that cycle, but I didn't go through a huge hormonal crash like the ones I'd experienced before. I left work a month later and two days later we discovered that I was pregnant. In June 2006 our son Tom was born."

Jeanie and Nick's case is a perfect illustration of the kind of story and outcome we have seen with many of our patients. Jeanie clearly needed medical help to diagnose and remove the fibroid that was affecting her chances of conceiving, but at the same time, the consultants that the couple visited saw nothing wrong with Nick's lifestyle, and didn't believe it could be affecting the quality of his sperm and their chances of conceiving. Acupuncture helped Jeanie to let go of much of the stress and anger she'd gone through while trying to conceive, and she was relieved to leave a stressful and unpleasant workplace. Nick made practical changes to his life, which ended up having a huge impact. In the end they didn't need to use IVF or ICSI to conceive.

Many patients attribute their improvement to the balancing nature of acupuncture treatment alone, but often their breakthrough involve a combination of help from hypnotherapy, counseling, IVF, surgery and even, like Nick and Jeanie, changing jobs or other lifestyle changes that they've made independently. Nothing is a definite cure and a complex problem can require many solutions. I hope that reading about their experience and the other stories in this book will help you to take an open-minded approach to that maze of options, and to see the many directions in which you can shift your attention to make any necessary change.

An Accidental Expert

When I started to practice Five-Element acupuncture I had no intention of specialising in infertility, but my work, which led to me becoming a "fertility expert" took off after I helped a single patient who wanted a cure for hay fever and got more than she bargained for.

At the time I was working for the NHS at Kings College Hospital part-time, mainly treating patients with HIV, AIDS and other immune-related disorders, and I'd set up a private practice in South London treating all kinds of symptoms including allergies, back pain and helping people quit smoking.

One of my first private patients, Maggie, was forty, married, worked as a solicitor and had one son, aged ten. After the first treatment she was delighted; her hay fever symptoms had disappeared completely and she was feeling surprisingly relaxed and just like her old self. I was delighted to get such a swift result too, and Maggie immediately referred three of her friends to my practice.

A month later Maggie made a new appointment, but this time she seemed even more ill than before. She wasn't very impressed by me. It was June and her hay fever had recurred, leaving her feeling exhausted and irritable. I gingerly gave her a second treatment, hoping it would do the trick this time. When she returned for a third session she was a different woman again: still exhausted, but she was absolutely ecstatic and could barely wait till she was in the treatment room to tell me her news; she was pregnant! She didn't tell me during her first consultation that she'd been trying to get pregnant for a second time for years and had been diagnosed as having "secondary infertility" five years previously.

Within weeks two of Maggie's friends that she had referred bounced into the treatment room with the same fanfare, also surprising me – neither of them had mentioned that they were trying to conceive, and I'd thought they'd come to me for stress-related problems. This flurry of surprise pregnancies caused a minor stir in South London and suddenly I was inundated with women who wanted the same magical instant-conception treatment. I found myself trying to explain that I wasn't treating infertility at all, but that my treatments were simply aimed at helping nature restore balance.

Let me explain the underlying philosophy of the treatments given, as the teachings are useful in helping you understand the importance of "balance" to your fertility.

The Nature of Balance

Five-Element acupuncture evolved in China more than five thousand years ago as a comprehensive system of medicine. This ancient culture had a profound understanding of the connection between the laws of nature and good health. The treatment was designed to balance the patient's system so that is was functioning optimally, which in turn eradicated disease and improved the quality of the patient's overall health including the effect of enhancing fertility. When the women in South London who came to me for treatment fell pregnant it really was an accident, or, more accurately, a side effect of a bigger change that had taken place in them.

The notion of not treating something in order to treat it is very Chinese. The Chinese love contradictions whereas we in the West want things to make sense, and so an understanding of ancient Chinese "thought" is helpful in making the connection between hay fever and irritable bowel syndrome or depression and infertility.

In the West it is relatively normal to wait until we're sick before we seek help. Preventative medicine is seen as alternative and rather unsatisfying because it fails to meet our results-orientated society. How much better it seems to be cured of cancer than prevent it in the first place. No one talks about the person that doesn't get sick, but we all love a story of someone overcoming a potentially fatal disease and the cast of heroes who swoop in to save the day. Surgeons in our culture are like Gods. In ancient China they were seen as butchers who stepped in when the physician had failed.

"Treating the person", a common expression in Five-Element Acupuncture, means making sure the body, mind and spirit of the person are functioning in a balanced and harmonious way. When everything is in order any symptoms will go away and we are well and can thrive.

A good analogy is of a house and how it provides the right environment for the family who lives there to be happy and healthy. The walls, windows and roof need to be well maintained and secure, the plumbing must carry fresh water throughout the house, the drains must carry away the waste. The boiler heats the water for radiators and the rooms ought to be decorated in a pleasant and stimulating way. By creating an environment that meets the needs of the family, and therefore providing a safe and happy home, it is more likely that within it there will be a balanced and pleasant existence free from sickness and pain. All of these factors – the heat, the water, the structure, the removal of waste, the décor – are interconnected, and if one is knocked out of sync the whole is affected. If the roof leaks, the walls will rot, the heating system will go on pumping out warm air that is lost to a draught and soon everyone in the house is sick.

I see a lot of people whose metaphorical houses are falling down around their ears, but who will swear blind that everything would be just fine as long as they could sort out their wheat intolerance or stop having hay fever or start having babies. The large majority of patients come for treatment because they've heard acupuncture is good for infertility, and they believe it will strengthen their reproductive system and help it to perform. To some extent that's true, but what the treatment really does is to reconnect the patient with something much more powerful than any conventional treatment or medication – their own innate intelligence and ability to find balance in order to return to optimum health. For some people this homeostatic response is so strong they rarely suffer from any symptoms at all - or if they do the problems are corrected almost immediately. The reason most of us seek help from a professional is that we have lost the ability to maintain balance and self-heal. It is also much easier for a third party to see what's going on with us, as by the time we reach our 30's we've been adjusting to minor symptoms and negative ways of being for so long that we find it all completely normal. This is particularly true of patients diagnosed with "unexplained infertility" where there are no obvious fertility related symptoms but more often than not many other minor problems.

The Five-Element practitioner has very particular skills to diagnose and treat imbalances, and can even detect a potential problem before any symptoms show. For example, if you came to me as a new patient and told me you have headaches, irregular periods and mild depression; I'd have to confess that your symptoms simply tell me you're out of balance and little else. The symptoms themselves don't say anything to me about how to treat you in the first instance, as they are simply alarm bells of distress saying there is something wrong, and it certainly would not be responsible of me to try to turn off the alarm bell before I've found the cause. There's no formula to do anything directly about those nagging superficial symptoms, instead the job is to head straight to the root and treat the cause.

The role of the practitioner is to care for the patient in the widest sense, to listen, to understand, to develop an authentic relationship, and then to interpret the entire experience through an intelligent and effective treatment that addresses the cause and will restore balance to help the person out of suffering.

The signs and signals we look for are not necessarily those that a western doctor would use for diagnosis, and as I said we do not treat symptoms directly when we find them. Where a doctor might provide an anti-histamine to stop a patient's eyes feeling itchy and their nose runny from hay fever, a Five-Element acupuncturist wants to uncover the true cause of why a person's system is out of balance and why it made them more vulnerable to illness that caused their hay fever symptoms or, as in Maggie's case, infertility.

"Traditional Chinese Medicine" or "TCM" is the most widespread type of acupuncture that you are likely to find in your town centre or on your high street, and it differs from Five-Element acupuncture. When Chairman Mao, the new Communist leader came to power in 1949, he needed a rudimentary health service to serve the growing Chinese population and get them back to work if they fell sick. This new regime shut down many educational institutions and drove practitioners of all styles of acupuncture out of work seeing the spiritual aspect of this medicine as elitist, superstitious and outdated. The Chinese people reacted greatly to this change, demanding acupuncture be reinstated, and so Mao, also under pressure to find mass medical health solutions, ordered the creation of a new style of acupuncture which was modernised, standardised and rolled out across the nation. It was a system that laid out recommended formulas and acupuncture points to use specifically for treating this or that syndrome or physical disorder. They kept the body map of points and the skills of pulse-taking previously used, but the core spiritual Taoist philosophy behind it was greatly reduced.

Many of the current studies into how acupuncture aids fertility look specifically at the treatment of organs and functions that directly relate to conception. This is then measured to evaluate the number of conceptions that result. For a Five-Element practitioner, the focus is not just on fertility and the intention is not to "make" couples conceive, in fact we can't; the best we can do is to help patients' systems find their way back to balance and when the factor that created imbalance in the first place is corrected or supported, their internal mechanism does the work.

The body, mind and spirit naturally seek balance, and the acupuncturist just facilitates this. For example, in a patient presenting with, let's say backache, a lack of confidence and infertility, these individual symptoms are not targeted one by one, but treated simultaneously as the internal homeostasis is restored and the core imbalance is addressed. I can only say the treatment has been truly successful if the patient ends the process feeling thoroughly well in their body, mind and spirit, symptoms addressed and with the appropriate energy to live their life to the full. That happy state may or may not include a baby.

A Philosophical Approach

So what is this ancient Chinese philosophy, and how is it useful to you?

"Taoist" philosophy sees the universe in paired terms: night and day, black and white, male and female. The ancient Chinese believed that heaven represented the father, earth represented the mother, and they, the humans, were the offspring of nature, created and maintained by these two parents. Everything in the world we see around us is the creation of the two primary forces of the mother and the father. You're probably familiar with the black and white symbol of yin and yang. Taoists see heaven as yang – the fatherly, lighter, and predominantly non-material, and earth as yin - the motherly, darker and predominantly material.

We humans live and experience everything between these two poles and we are sustained throughout our lives by each heavenly breath we inspire from our "father", and every earthly morsel of food we ingest from our "mother". We're a combination of material and nonmaterial, and our challenge is to balance the two, and if we're successful we will, in theory, thrive, reproduce, and survive for a hundred years! When we fail to maintain that balance, we get sick, and as long as we are sick our symptoms remind us we've lost that balance.

The dynamic coming together and reaction of the two poles of nonmaterial and material, heaven and earth, permanent and impermanent, also produces the five elements: wood, fire, earth, metal and water; our world. Everything in existence is made up of a compound of these elements found in nature, and human beings are no exception. We exist as all five, and the balance of those elements is unique to each of us, and can also vary by the day or even the hour. To return to my earlier analogy, the elements are the impermanent components of the house – the heating, the walls, the roof, and so on – it's what makes us unique, and is our personality and is in a constant state of change. The permanent "self" at our core is the origin or foundation of the house. That "self" is who we really are and is constant - our whole potential and the five elements enable that potential to come to fruition, as an outer projected impermanent structure – the house.

Each of the five elements has certain qualities and associations that can be related to every aspect of the human experience. They shape our physical bodies, internal organs and systems, organise our thoughts and fuel our feelings and give our life form; they also make babies.

For you to be in the fullness of who you are as a unique human being, and have the capacity to express yourself and reproduce, all five elements need to be present, engaged, and working together to maintain a balanced relationship with one another. In this healthy state, all the elements maintain equilibrium, adjusting for each new situation life presents and then settling back into place, or reconfiguring ready to tackle each fresh challenge. So, on an emotional level, if someone does something against you, the wood element reacts and you can be appropriately angry; if someone says something funny, the fire element responds and you can be appropriately amused; if you are in need, the earth element provides and you feel appropriately nourished; if you experience loss, the metal element connects and helps you appropriately grieve; and if you are being chased and feel fear, the water element surges and you can run for your life! When you respond spontaneously and appropriately, you can roll with the constant flux of life. Making a baby is no different; each of the Five Elements having an assigned role and responding to the intricate process of creating new life. A natural homeostasis operates in everything, a universal life force working in us all to guide us through the turbulence of the human experience and back to a harmonious state, which survives us, even when we die.

However, part of the challenge of being a human being is that each person has a flaw, a kind of Achilles heel or imbalance rooted in one of the five elements. It's a default setting that we all have and consistent with the dualistic nature of life, and is the original cause of all imbalances in us.

Professor J .R Worsley, who was one of my teachers and credited with bringing Five-Element acupuncture to the West, believed and taught that every human being has one original elemental imbalance, or "causative factor" that remains constant throughout his or her life regardless of the current state of health. We can easily slip with the pressures of life, and any, or all of the elements can suffer as a result. However this slip will always be rooted in the person's weakest element, and all problems, mental, physical and spiritual stem from this place. This is a significant starting point when looking for the causes of unexplained infertility.

For the Five-Element acupuncturist of Worsley's tradition, identifying that element is essential to treating a patient successfully. It is the key to getting that person back on track. For our purposes, however, an understanding of each of the elements and how they function in you will provide you with an awareness of whether you are in balance, and more importantly, if and how you are not. By having this greater insight into how you function and behave, any necessary change becomes an immediate possibility, in turn positively shifting your general health and your fertility. You already have an intimate relationship with the five elements needed for balance and health; it's now simply a matter of ensuring they all function as one.

Finding Balance

So how do we know if one, or all of the elements are imbalanced in us?

The moment any one of the Five Elements becomes distressed it immediately sends out a signal asking for help, and this will be apparent in many different ways. A Five-Element acupuncturist is looking for and diagnoses a patient's "causative factor" the primary elemental imbalance, by paying attention to a colour that shows on the face around the eyes, a sound in their voice, an odour and a predominant emotion. For example a patient with a "causative factor" in the earth element, the colour will be yellow, have a sing-song sound, smell slightly sweet and crave understanding and sympathy. A patient with a "causative factor" in the wood element, the colour will be green, have a clipped sound, smell rancid and will appear frustrated and angry. As human faces, voices, odours and emotions come in every variation; this might seem a rather curious statement to make – how could the whole of mankind possibly appear in just five ways that relate to a distress call in one of the five elements?

The answer is that these distress signals underlie all the other factors, because it's nature's way of alerting us to the cause of the problem; to the very skilled diagnostician - it is obvious. It can take years to develop an expertise in recognising these signs in others, but we do all have that ability, whether we are acupuncturists or not. The more we awaken from our slumber and pay attention to what nature is telling us, this kind of information becomes more obvious all the time.

We react all the time to smells in the street even if only unconsciously, crossing the road without thinking, or suddenly feeling hungry because of a whiff of fresh bread from a bakery. We know when someone in front of us in a queue is agitated or threatening. Think of the way that a mother can catch a tone in her child's voice before more than a dozen words are said on the phone and know instantly that he or she is sad, excited, angry or in need. Parents watch their children, their lovers and partners the whole time. If we pick up the slightest change in their complexions and smells, we react. It doesn't matter what they say, because we have already sensed the direction their feelings have taken. If you took away our senses and left only words, no one would have a clue what was going on.

If I walk into a room with a new patient waiting, it's always very exciting as there will be one predominant odour in the room that is being produced by one of the elements that will speak to me to help me make a diagnosis, and is nothing to do with sweat, perfume or unwashed clothes. To the expert nose, someone who is very imbalanced can give off an element odour so strong that it's quite disconcerting at first.

We might not consciously think about it, but we do register everything at some primitive, instinctive level and we certainly use these natural skills for our own survival. Five-Element diagnosis draws heavily on these skills, and it can take a practitioner a long time to learn to use them consciously and accurately, but for the layperson, becoming conscious and being able to read this coded information about our self and others is essential at a time of sickness and confusion. Understanding what nature is telling us, not only provides the answers to what we are looking for, but also brings a sense of calm; our tolerance and compassion for ourself and others enhanced, where normally these signs could be ignored or jar us and grate on our nerves.

As I go on with the explanation of Taoist Five-Element philosophy, you will see that the Chinese recognised that everything in life is interconnected, and when one part of the whole is affected this will in turn affect everything else, as in the description of the house in the first chapter.

The Five Elements correspond to five Chinese seasons: wood in spring, fire in summer, earth in late summer, metal in autumn and water in winter. Each season, like each element, is a manifestation of nature as it goes through its cycle of growth in spring, flowering in summer, harvest in late summer, decomposition in autumn and regeneration in winter: five stages of one year.

The elements are also responsible for the creation and maintenance of the organs, body parts and functions of the human body, because we are part of nature and our physical structure mirrors that of our external world. This microcosm of the human body is scaled up to nature as a whole, like a larger but otherwise identical Russian doll. For example, in the same way that the convection cycle draws water from rivers, lakes and oceans to form clouds which descend on mountains and back down to earth as nourishing rain, so our kidneys and bladder control the water in our body, cleansing, lubricating and providing enormous reserves of flowing energy.

Chinese medicine differs greatly from Western medicine in the way it sees the purpose and role of our internal organs and functions. In the Chinese system the organs and functions, also known as "Officials", have specific responsibilities that not only deal with the physical, but every aspect of being human. Taking the previous example of the kidneys and bladder, not only do these two "Officials" process fluids but also govern our drive and ambition, our ability to find stillness and peace, and our instinct to survive - to name but a few. Unlike the Western approach of compartmentalising organ functions and diseases, the Chinese system sees the interconnectedness and the complex internal relationships of our organs and functions extend to every aspect of our overall health. This is essential to grasp when looking at the possible causes of infertility and what is required to conceive. We not only take in air, water and food from the outside world but also vast quantities of information and life experience that affects us both positively and negatively, and the organs and functions each have a role in processing those influxes.

Most infertility treatments, both conventional and alternative, tend to concentrate on the reproductive organs and the endocrine system that governs our hormones, without considering the other organs and systems which underpin, supply and support them.

Each and every one of the five elements are essential for creating the right conditions for successful conception and pregnancy, for example: wood for regulation of the menstrual cycle, the male erection and the growth of the foetus, fire for passion and sexual activity, temperature regulation, the warming of the womb and cooling the testicles, earth to nourish the blood, build the uterine lining and feed the developing baby, metal to provide quality air, essential trace elements and release the waste, water for the power of creation, regulation of the hormonal flow and maturation of healthy eggs and sperm.

As you read on and learn more about the elements and their associated organs and functions it may seem that there are some surprising omissions – brain, for example, or uterus – but these fall under the category of secondary or "extraordinary" organs in the Chinese system. As this is a guide to baby-making rather than a textbook on Five-Element acupuncture, I will only describe the primary organs and functions directly associated with each of the elements, their defined roles and how they contribute to a balanced state of being and how when they are out of balance they will produce symptoms and negatively affect your fertility. I will also give a case study to show how when an element is in distress it can be detrimental to the person in many ways.

Thankfully, there is no expectation or need for you to diagnose yourself from what you read as you will recognise yourself in all the elements, some more than others, but the descriptions of the elements and the characters in the case studies will help you recognise where you might be out of balance and struggle and possibly need to make changes - and maybe even ask for help.

The Five Elements

Wood

The wood element is associated with the season spring. The Five-Element acupuncturist's diagnosis for a person with an imbalance in this element is the colour green showing in the face, the odour given off is rancid, the timbre to the voice is a shout or a tight, clipped sound, and the primary emotion experienced with this element is anger or a lack of anger. This might seem like a strange association to make, but you have to recognise spring as a time when everything comes alive and begins to expand and grow. There is a sense of relief and freedom as vegetation that died or went underground in winter grows again, and new animals are born. Just when most of nature seemed to be dead it is revealed to have been only sleeping all along. For us this also means everything awakens and now feels possible, and so it's a time to make plans and employ strategies to move on.

Now imagine being a seed underground ready to burst forth; a paving slab is placed on top of the ground above you and stops your action and all your potential. How would you feel? The Chinese pictogram for "anger" is of a tree growing in a box; something that is not allowed to grow healthily in an unchecked fashion. When you have a primary imbalance in the wood element you have a feeling of being restricted, frustrated and angry: either you have an abnormal amount of anger which comes shooting out of you at the vaguest provocation, or else you feel defeated, devoid of the assertiveness which could help you move and change, and yet under this seemingly passive state you feel angry, resigned and depressed. We tend to see anger as a negative emotion, and it can be when it is not used well, or flares up strongly, but it's also a driving force; if we do not grow and develop as nature intends, the whole cycle of life can feel like it ends before it begins.

Wood is seen as holding the plan of life and provides the strategy for all action. It provides the direction and focus for what the body, mind and spirit is going to do and how it's going to keep going and survive. Because our primary job as human beings is to be who we are and bring the uniqueness and fullness of ourselves into the world, we need this element to give us the vision and clarity so that we can see ourselves and our situation clearly enough to take action as our life unfolds. If something gets in our way, we need the flexibility to either engage and make change or find a way to adapt rather than simply becoming blocked and stuck.

Wood's associated organs are the gall bladder and the liver. The Chinese system maintains that physiologically the gall bladder produces and secretes bile to assist in the break down of fats, which helps with the digestive process. Digesting food continues through the digestive tract and eventually transforms into nourishing blood entering the liver, which further purifies and passes this life giving substance on to the rest of the body.

Five-Element acupuncture ascribes a further role to the gall bladder and liver of organising and directing all the body's other organs. Any action that materialises in life requires a plan and a decision. Our immune system can't fight off infections if it doesn't strike and attack a foreign body; the stomach cannot digest the food if it doesn't have the ability to balance digestive juices, and our tendons and ligaments cannot bend and stretch without the flexibility of wood's great plan. All kinds of symptoms such as stomach ulcers, menstrual cramps, irritable bowel syndrome, and irregular menstruation can result when the wood element no longer functions correctly.

The bottled up frustration often seen with an imbalance in wood also leads to physical symptoms like tension pain from wrought-up muscles, RSI, headaches, eye problems, weak nails, poor digestion and even breathing problems.

I often am alerted to diagnose a patient with a wood imbalance as soon as I walk into the waiting room at the clinic. The first hint: although subtle, a look as though they are furious with me, and then all smiles and politeness on greeting, and then they almost crush my hand as I shake it. On entering the treatment room they don't just place their bag down - they throw it down. Others are self-effacing to the point of timidity, but if you hit the wrong subject they're primed to explode. Patients who come for treatment are often not aware that the way they feel or behave is in any way strange – it's all they know. If you ask if they are frustrated or angry they will look surprised and vehemently deny it, or blame their mood on others around them who are inconsiderate or annoying.

There's nothing wrong with them, you understand, it's just everyone else!

Wood: A case study

"They told me there was parking nearby – and there's not!" Ruby shot at me. Taken aback and confused by the soft gentle hand in mine, I immediately pulled away, apologised for the misinformation and indicated the direction of my treatment room.

Ruby was 32, a striking looking woman with piercing eyes and the longest floating limbs I've ever seen. As she climbed the stairs in front of me I was mesmerised by her graceful and fluid flight, her body lifting step by step; each movement seemed choreographed to the finest detail. Once settled in the room she immediately opened the Consultation. "I need to be pregnant by the end of June", she told me staring. "Otherwise I will wait until next year... I am sure you can help me". Her mouth smiled but her eyes did not warm or blink – the gauntlet was thrown.

She'd been with her husband for five years and had stopped taking the contraceptive pill a year prior to coming to me. Her periods were regular and, as she proudly told me, were running like a "Swiss clock". She was surprised and disappointed that she had not already conceived but put it down to a very erratic sex life due to both their work commitments. Her only other complaint was tension in her jaw and headaches at the back of her head. Her body was an unusual combination of super flexibility noticeable when I lifted her arm, which floated off the treatment couch, and absolute tension in her neck when she attempted to move her head from side to side.

As I explained how treatment works and what she

could expect, I couldn't help notice her glancing up to the ceiling and hear 'tut' fire-like small pellets from her tightly pursed lips. I was clearly irritating her and anything other than the essentials of treatment was going to cause her stress.

Ruby came for treatment every Tuesday morning at 8.15am. She was never late and I made sure to finish on time; she was a very busy woman. During a typical treatment, prior to inserting a needle, I warm the area over the acupuncture point with Moxa, a Chinese herb that is placed and burnt over the skin. Rather than tell me when she felt the pleasant warming sensation as guided, Ruby would wait for it to burn and then swear at me.

In spite of any misgivings I may have had at first, we worked well together and she responded to treatment. Her neck relaxed, her headaches cleared and on treatment six she arrived at 8.18am. Now I knew I was getting somewhere. Most importantly, during one session when she was lying on the treatment couch she revealed to me that a recurrent nightmare she had had since childhood had suddenly changed. She told me the story.

When Ruby was 14 her older brother Adam was killed in a car crash. They had been inseparable their whole lives and now without warning she was an only child. As she told me about Adam and his death she cried and gripped me so tightly the blood was forced out of my hand and into my fingertips. Until recently, since that day she had this same short dream every night. They would be walking through a field she knew

49

from childhood and suddenly without warning her brother would run off with a group of his friends and be gone, no longer wanting to be seen with her – he was now too grown up. The feelings of hurt and anger from this apparent rejection would haunt her nightly and she would wake with tears running down her face.

Ruby began to relax with me as she recounted her dream, and even more so as she reported that since her acupuncture treatment started Adam would appear in her dream, but rather than run away, he would stay.

Ruby conceived bang on schedule. That wasn't changing, but the charge around her did, to a softer, easier, more at peace Ruby.

Fire

Fire is the element of summer. Unlike wood, water, earth and metal, it is associated with not only two organs – the heart and small intestine – but also two functions which don't have a physical form and which are called "circulation-sex" and "three heater".

The heart was seen by the ancient Chinese as our direct connection with Heaven and was considered the most important organ in the body as it pumps blood and life to every cell, a unifying action. The heart is the seat of passion and love, sending out blood unconditionally to every cell in the body to maintain life. The small intestine known as the "separator of pure from impure", supports the heart by filtering out impurities and the detritus and irrelevance of daily life and leaving the heart free to receive the "mandate of heaven". The "three heater" maintains and regulates temperature by keeping the passageways clear and acts like a thermostat, and "circulation-sex" is, as the name suggests, responsible for the circulatory system and for our passion and sexual activity. We recognise this as when we are aroused, blood is sent to our genitals and to our lips, making them fuller and more sensitive. Symbolically, the "three heater" and "circulation-sex" open our heart, our inner private self to our outer world and the hearts of others.

So what can happen when you have an imbalance in the fire element? The odour is that of burnt or scorched material.   When the fire element is functioning properly, it will hold you on an even keel with an appropriate level of joy, like the comforting warmth of a farmhouse Aga. People with an imbalance in fire can "overheat", be inappropriately exuberant and demanding, and almost hysterically happy about everything, even if it's sad. The flipped version is the person who cannot find joy in almost anything, and who withdraws from company and seems indifferent and cold. You can recognise someone with an imbalance in the fire element by the sound in their voice - it either has a relentless laugh to it, or it's sapped of emotion and flat. The colour seen on the face at each side of the patient's eyes is a reflection of that too; grey if there is too little fire, and red if there is too much.

When fire is functioning well, we unconditionally generate love for ourself and for others and feel safe at home in our self and out in the world. We know when to open and when to close; we are at our fullest potential as individuals. However, when the fire is struggling or almost burnt out we feel vulnerable and defenceless, and lose our ability to communicate properly and openly with others, walking down the street with our eyes cast down to avoid other people's attention. People with a causative factor in fire can be quick to abandon their friends who have hurt or offended them, even if to an outsider, the initial conflict doesn't seem so grave.

This inconsistency in social interaction can lead to leaping into friendships and being desperate to be best friends straight away, at times intruding into the other person's life; there seems to be a need to almost engulf that person. They lack the subtle skill of healthy boundaries and often blow hot and cold socially and though their pathology is more apparent in emotional issues, it also might manifest in physical symptoms; circulation problems, heart palpitations, boils and other indicators that all is not well.

Fire: A case study

I have to confess I can't remember the name of this patient, as privately I affectionately called him "The Laughing Salesman". About fifteen years ago I was employed by companies to go to their offices once a week and treat eight or so of their employees. The laughing salesman was one of my patients. I always knew when he was on his way as I could hear him whistling and chirping to himself as he came down the long echoing corridor to the treatment room. Then he'd rap on the door in some jokey rhythm, and he'd fly into the room, make a quip, laugh, start pulling off his clothes immediately, pull a face and bellow with laughter once more. Everything he did had to be a joke. He couldn't help himself. He couldn't take anything seriously. The banter was relentless, and after a while it really began to grate on me. As he sat on the couch in his underpants and socks, he swung his legs back and forth like a little boy struggling to stay still.

He was extremely good at his job as a salesman with that ceaseless energy. He'd come in at 5am, drink buckets of coffee and challenge all the younger guys to a squash match in the company gym. The office was large enough for him to bounce from desk to desk telling his jokes without exasperating too many people, but you couldn't have contained him in a smaller set up with a small group of people – they would have killed themselves or quit after a week or two.

It was another story for his wife of course, who, it sounded to me, was exhausted with the effort of keeping up with him. Once he cheerily told me that she'd asked him to book a nice relaxing holiday at a good hotel by the sea, and he'd decided that that couldn't possibly be what she wanted – far too boring – and hired a camper van for them to drive around America instead. Poor Sheila.

He was only in his mid-thirties but his face was scarlet, his blood pressure was soaring and his body was permanently hot. It was as though he'd never matured properly; he was just cooking the whole time and never finished. He also had a low sperm count, and he and his wife were having difficulty conceiving.

Working with him was an uphill struggle for me and it took a very long time to see palpable results. It was a challenge to get him to just feel neutral about something, without laughing manically and turning it into a joke. In our culture we place a high value on joy and being "up" and try to avoid feelings that are negative or low, but too much of any emotion is bad – everything must be given its balanced expression.

Gradually, notch by notch he calmed down. His high colouring began to fade and I no longer felt like I was touching a hot plate when I checked his pulse. I tried to encourage him to do something he liked, like swimming, rather than thrash around the squash court out of sheer competitiveness. He went from an almost total lack of self-awareness to being able to have meaningful conversations. After many months of treatment and lifestyle changes, he reported that his wife had conceived and he was going to be a dad.

Earth

The Chinese separate summer into two parts, and Earth is the element connected to the harvest season of late summer. The crops are gathered and brought into granaries for winter storage. Metaphorically, you can see its connection with the associated organs; the stomach, which also takes in food and resources, and the spleen, which turns that food into energy and nourishment and stores the extra as fat for future needs. The spleen is considered the Minister for Transport, moving everything along that we take in – from ideas, to food, to all of our emotions.

The colour is yellow, the smell is sweet, an oaty one of fermentation, and the sound in the voice is a sing-song, a bit like a lullaby, as when a mother speaks to a child. People with a causative factor in earth seem to be primarily caught up in nurturing and sympathy (or the lack of). The element is responsible for the way we care or look after ourselves and others around us, and monitors our nourishment on all levels. Have our guests got enough to eat? Are there good books to read on the shelf? Are we all going to have the most comfortable seats on the flight? It's a kind of circular relationship of giving things out and taking them in, of interaction with our environment.

Some people whose earth element is in trouble are often curled inward and caught in their own world of feeling sorry for themselves. They believe they don't have enough. They ask for sympathy but reject it when they receive it because they simply can't "take it in" and "process" it. It's as though they think they have no choice but to function without any true interaction with others, while at the same time it's obvious to a bystander that they need their help. It's a little like seeing an anorexic so obviously starving but refusing to take food when it is offered.

Equally the reverse can be true. People desperate to provide an environment that they believe will make you happy, and by default please them, hurl themselves into an "earth mother" role by doling out provisions, understanding and sympathy like a tsunami that is more likely to swamp you rather than help you. If you have a headache they know exactly how it feels because they had one, only it was worse. You might just be chatting and telling them about your recent trip to the shops where you forgot your money but the intensity of their attention to your story and the resulting sympathy seems completely inappropriate. They have no guard or brake when it comes to giving "care" and just go on giving it out and piling it up.

Physically, the knock-on effect of an imbalance in this element is often seen in digestive and metabolism problems. A person seems ravenous and constantly eats but never gains weight because they can't process food properly, or else they don't known when to stop as no matter how much they eat they never feel satisfied. Feeling this emptiness and fearing there will be no more food in the future, they keep on eating and of course their body packs on fat. Nothing is being processed properly, so they are often groggy physically and mentally, and because they are continually taking everything on board, very little is getting processed and sent to the right place. Other symptoms include gastric reflux, bloating and flatulence - even recurrent miscarriage. When earth is balanced however, a person knows exactly how much food to eat or information to process or emotion to absorb, and certainly when to stop.

Case Study: Earth

When I think of a great example of somebody with an imbalance in the earth element, my lovely patient Sarah springs to mind. She was in her late thirties when she came to see me for help. She'd been mistress to a man twenty years older than her for nearly two decades who already had adult children, and now she wanted to have a baby with him.

She said that several doctors had told her she was anorexic, and she was indeed very, very thin, but I didn't think this diagnosis or label was helpful or true – she was neither interested nor disinterested in food, she just simply appeared not to care if she fed herself or not. Sometimes she ate a lot, and other times she went without food for days and didn't notice. Sometimes she couldn't even remember the last time she ate. She also hadn't had a period for years.

This pattern of not knowing what was good for her was repeated throughout her life. Her life as a whole – as mistress to this man – didn't make much sense. Although she claimed she was very happy in this situation she didn't convince me by how she described her life whenever we met. She gave enormously to him and everyone around her but seemed to receive very little in return. She'd earlier had a second affair with another man and fallen pregnant, but decided against having the baby at a very late stage because she didn't think she was sure she wanted to be a mother after all. She would regularly visit friends in the country at weekends but almost always describe the experience as a waste of her time as she ended up doing all the housework. She was strangely undemanding of me and of the people around her, and yet from the stories she would tell me it was clear she was ultimately left feeling empty and alone. I often wondered what she really thought of her appointments with me. From what I could tell she didn't seem to know what she wanted from life, other than a child.

At our sessions together, in addition to using needles, I used a very prescriptive form of support by giving her homework, asking her to eat breakfast every day for three months, and to keep a diary of this in order to keep her focussed on the task. It felt like teaching a child. As treatment progressed over many months, slowly she opened up and began to talk about her relationship, her friends and her work and to see what she actually got from these different areas of her life. She started to recognise the people and activities that gave her a feeling of satisfaction and joy and most strikingly began avoiding the people that took her for granted and took advantage of her very sweet and giving nature.

Her periods didn't restart and she didn't gain much weight, but she did conceive again and carried the baby to full term. Her doctor who had threatened to forcibly send her to a treatment centre for anorexia was amazed at how this stick thin woman could carry a pregnancy with such ease and grace and produce a healthy well-nourished baby girl.

Having the baby seemed to further engage Sarah in the material world. She transformed completely as she fully embraced motherhood and now on weekend visits to the country, rather than take the role of serving her fellow house- guests, she developed the art of asking for and receiving help and properly integrating into the group.

Metal

Metal is the element associated with autumn, the point in the annual cycle where plants are dying and everything is sinking back into the earth. The harvest is stored and anything we don't need should now be swept away. What's left is a very pure, mineral essence, stripped down and compressed much like the gold and diamonds we find buried deep within the earth. When this element is in distress, the colour we see in a person's face is white, and the timbre of the voice is a weep; like gentle sobbing. The smell is of something rotten, as though the person's pores aren't opening properly and clearing away the waste.

Metal equates to the value of things: our inner and outer riches. The associated organs are the lungs and the colon. The lungs draw in fresh air and represent our ability to take life in, the breath of heaven, keeping us alive and connected. The colon is connected to earth and death and a final rotting down, and of course, the removal of all waste. When metal is in balance we take in freshness and discard the nonsense and extraneous detail of our everyday lives. We know who we are and what the value of our unique role is in the world, and we also have a natural mechanism to rid ourselves of doubt or derision. Preserving that purity is essential to our well being, whether it's emptying the rubbish bins or letting go of something hurtful that someone has said to us.

Not surprisingly, people with a metal imbalance can feel like they live under a dark cloud or are buried in the clutter (often literally) and minutiae of everyday life. They flap around hopelessly not knowing what they're looking for or how to find it. Physically they have a tendency towards symptoms where waste is not removed and can have issues with constipation and diarrhea. In Chinese medicine the skin is considered the third lung that breathes and connects with the outside world, and so they can struggle with eczema and psoriasis, have problems breathing fully and deeply, and often suffer from asthma or recurrent bronchial infections.

The primary emotion is grief, as though one is living in a void, or caught in a past memory of someone or something instead of moving on in the present. It becomes really hard to connect with the here and now and so the person often looks longingly to another time. A lot of people with a metal imbalance are weighed down with the sense that they are not good enough and that gets in the way of them achieving the task that's right before them. Old baggage and a lack of fresh inspiration drag them down and distracts them. They're always looking for something better because they cannot relish the good that's here right now. They find it hard to find the value in almost anything and so they become critical of themselves and others. Nothing ever feels good enough. This makes them dismissive of themselves and others. When it comes to fertility even an embryo can be dismissed when this element is out of balance.

Struggling to take in and entertain new ideas makes them cynical, and if you've ever come across that "yeah, life's pointless but let's get on with it anyway" attitude you may have possibly met someone whose metal is sick. Sadly for them, their focus is on their own bad qualities and those of everyone around them.

Case Study: Metal

Virginia was at least twenty minutes late for her first appointment, and arrived with a list of excuses that simply didn't add up. Her designer shirt was splattered with grease; she had chewed nails and severely laddered tights. As she searched for her medical records in her large battered handbag she revealed among other things, an empty yoghurt carton and a screwdriver.

She smelt musty. Even though she wore expensive clothes she looked slightly mucky, and the stories that poured out of her mouth like diarrhea were full of gossip, resentment and blame. My experience of her was that everything about her was rotting and bitter, as if she was completely overwhelmed by her own negativity.

Virginia was 39 and had been with her partner for just over five years. They had never used contraception, had never conceived, and Virginia had given up hope that she would ever get pregnant. She had come for treatment because a friend had insisted that she try. She reluctantly answered my questions but was not willing to entertain any helpful suggestions from me about diet, exercise and so forth, all of which were immediately dismissed. She seemed to have lost faith in everything.

This "experience" of Virginia in the room told me everything I needed to know about how I could help her. No doctor, blood tests or scans, not even Virginia herself could have revealed in words so much to me as she did in these first few minutes. She had been diagnosed by her consultant as having unexplained infertility, but the truth was that she was in a terrible state; she was emotionally and physically a mess.

My job with Virginia was a simple one. I had to help her clean up her act and bring back a sense of hope. Acupuncture treatment is unbelievably effective in a situation like this. There is an acupuncture point on the lung channel called "Meridian Gutter" that when needled acts like a broom which brushes through the meridians (the energy pathways) clearing the rubbish from the gutters, the darkened corners, and brings fresh air and space to every part of the body and mind to reveal the spirit. It sounds bizarre, but with patients like Virginia it is nothing short of miraculous.

After this treatment Virginia was transformed. She arrived on time to her next appointment and described herself as feeling as if an enormous weight had been lifted off her chest and shoulders. She had spent the whole week cleaning her house without any suggestion from me, her bowels had started to become regular and her joint pain had eased up so much that she didn't need the medication she had been prescribed. She even talked about the possibility of becoming a mother.

After a year she conceived naturally and had a very happy and healthy pregnancy ending with the birth of her daughter, Lily.

Water

Winter is the season of the water element and is the time when everything in nature is still and quiet. Energy and power is hidden and low. Someone with a water imbalance reveals a blue colour to their face, and the sound in their voice is a groan, a weak, strained and monotonous sound, or a relentless deluge of sound. The odour is putrid like stagnating water which hasn't been moving as it should. Winter was historically a challenging and terrifying time for people as they waited and hoped that their supplies would last until the spring, and the associated emotion is fear.

We all need fear to survive. Fear alerts us to danger and gives us the reflex to stay safe by giving us the energy for "fight-or-flight". Something as simple as crossing the road requires an appropriate amount of fear, healthy caution helps us sum up the risks before we stride out. This automatic reflex that most of us take for granted is often lacking in people with an imbalance in water. These patients are sometimes takers of huge risks, as they can't calculate whether they should be cautious or not. Equally people with a water imbalance can swing the other way and become abnormally afraid of everyday life. They feel nervous of using new machinery in case something goes wrong, convince themselves that the approaching storm will destroy their home and even something as simple as coming for an appointment with someone like me can turn into a nail biting cliff hanger affair. Many times I have jumped myself on approaching a patient for the first time, as they leap to their feet, eyes wide open. They often develop all kinds of phobias as the underlying inherent fear is projected out on to all kinds of situations.

The bladder and the kidneys are the associated organs to water. In Chinese medicine the bladder has a much greater importance than we give it credit for in Western medicine. The bladder doesn't just act as a container for wastewater; it also assesses the balance of fluid in the whole body and ensures that the proper reserves are held in the right physical location for the right amount of time. For example, we need fluids at our eyes for lubrication and tears and sexual secretions for sexual intercourse. The fluidity and ease of movement throughout the entire system is dependent on the function of the bladder. The kidneys control and distribute the fluids and are responsible for the base, underlying power and energy of the whole body. The kidneys hold our very essence, the core of who we are and give us our deepest sense of self; our identity in form.

Water is the element that controls the endocrine system, instrumental in the regulation of our moods, growth and development and importantly, sexual function and fertility. People with a causative factor in water often suffer from a low libido and general lethargy, at times even presenting a history of recurrent miscarriage and their energy lacking the power and vitality to cope with the strain. Kidney problems affect the distribution of fluids – resulting in symptoms like oedema, swollen ankles or dry eyes. People whose water element and energy has become deficient will experience symptoms of cold and stagnation – feeling inert and clammy to the touch.

Case Study: Water

The first consultation with Jen was extraordinary. As she told me about her failure to conceive she became absolutely hysterical. I have seen people devastated or depressed about not getting pregnant, but this woman was wild, crying and shouting at me.

In the past I used to work more slowly and sit with people's various ways of communicating, but I've become increasingly inclined to cut to the chase when it is obvious that the behaviour is so inappropriate it will slow down the process of working together to get them well. I tried to bring her attention to how bizarre this display of emotion was to me and that we needed to slow down and take time to get some perspective. She fought at first, but in the course of the next hour and a half she calmed down and started talking coherently. This initial display however had told me all I needed to know in terms of how to help her.

Jen and her husband already had a child and were trying for a second. He was frequently away on long work trips, and she preferred to stay on her own with her daughter, rarely socialising. She was living a bizarre, cloistered life in her pretty house with a state of the art security system because she was terrified of the dangers of the world and other people. If her daughter so much as toddled towards the staircase she would pounce on her, screaming, and terrify the child. She existed in a constant state of fear, and had come to think it was perfectly normal. She worried about crime, child abductions, any threat she could dream up. She told me – and herself – that she wasn't a people person and that was why she didn't see many people, but all I could see was a personal security system every bit as defensive as the one on her home. If you met her in everyday life, you probably wouldn't have noticed this imbalance, because she had quite simply structured her life in a manner that allowed her to avoid, for the most part, dealing with the outside world. It was all damage limitation, rather than facing up to the risks and benefits of the real world.

Physically, not surprisingly, she was wrung out with adrenalin. She threw herself into the future and imagined her little girl as an only child, alone and in danger without a sibling. It was almost as if this second baby was imagined as a sort of donor child to help the first child live. It had never occurred to Jen that at base she was trying to protect herself from the world of fear she'd created.

The first task I gave her was to get in contact with two old friends she hadn't seen for a long time. I'd been brusque in the first consultation, but equally she was quick to knock down the old walls of fear she'd built. She was genuinely shocked when she reflected and realised how strangely she'd been behaving. On the back of this awareness she became more and more at peace in herself, her desperation for a second child transformed into being simply hopeful. She understood that her daughter would be in no greater danger than any other child as a result of being an only child.

All of these case studies demonstrate how one imbalanced element can greatly affect and dominate a person's life and health and cause all kinds of seemingly unrelated problems. The way that we "are" and behave is frequently dismissed or judged as just part of our "personality" rather than seen as useful information about something far more interesting, how we have become unbalanced. We do it to ourselves all the time with language and excuses like "I can't help it – it's just the way I am", or "I'm just moody, like everyone in my family", or "I'm a very sensitive person". Worse still, we exacerbate the problem by judging others and putting them in a box when we see repetitive behavior or a certain trait, and label them as "touchy", "irritable", "sympathetic", "nervy", or "great fun". Whatever the label, good or bad, it really doesn't matter - it's still just a label for a state that a person has got stuck in – and most importantly is unknowingly crying out for help. There is no such thing as an "irritable person", an "anxious person", or a "fearful person". We are simply describing someone with certain thoughts, feelings and behaviours that are stuck, unable to move appropriately and unwittingly causing all kinds of knock-on effects, including problems with fertility.

The Five Element model teaches us to pay close attention to the part of us that is unbalanced and sick, to become aware of the cause, and do all we can to support that weakness. Whether this is done through acupuncture, lifestyle changes, breaking old habits, or thinking differently; by virtue of the interrelationships between all the elements, any kind of change you make for the better will immediately improve your whole system. Successful conception and pregnancy is always a team effort involving the five elements equally; ask any team coach the secret of success, and he or she will always tell you "support your weakest player'.

Spirit

A few years ago I was treating a woman called Geraldine who aged 39 had decided to have a child on her own. She was having IUI with donor sperm at a Harley Street Clinic and had come for a "boost", but it rapidly became clear that she suffered deeply from depression and many small physical complaints. She told me that her younger sister had died when she was four, and her memories of her parents' grief and withdrawal had affected her deeply. She felt they lost their real connection to her at that time. By her teenage years, she was on course for what she called "dysfunctional relationships" with men who were chaotic and reckless, and she'd started to abuse both alcohol and drugs.

She said that every morning, for as long as she could remember, she'd woken up with a sense of dread so acute that it was like getting a boot in the stomach. By the time she came to see me she had been through Alcoholics Anonymous and Narcotics Anonymous and was on the straight and narrow, but she was also desperately lonely. She'd lost a lot of friends in giving up alcohol, and was ticking every symptom for clinical depression.

For us humans to function at our optimum and benefit from good overall health, we need the relationship between our body, mind and spirit to be "balanced". Feeling physically unwell, or emotionally flat, depressed, hopeless or stuck, or any one of the negative experiences we label as sickness or depression, in my experience, is usually the result of our inability to access our "spirit", and enjoy the miracle of being alive.

When I first considered training in Five-Element acupuncture, although fascinated by the theory of the Five Elements per se, I was not completely convinced by the notion or relevance of "spirit". It seemed to me at the time a very unnecessary "airy-fairy" adjunct to this system of medicine and its relevance to health and healing as a whole. In fact, after three long years of study I only fully appreciated the power of "spirit" as a key to real success when I started to work with patients and witnessed many surprising outcomes. Although the notion of spirit as an active ingredient in helping you conceive may seem fanciful and mystical, once properly understood, I am sure it will start to feel surprisingly familiar and logical, and most importantly transformational. Professor J.R. Worsley helps demystify this idea of "spirit" in this extract from his book "Is Acupuncture for You?".

"A lot of people feel uncomfortable when you mention the word "spirit". They think you are talking about some mystical entity, or are about to embark on some form of religious crusade. Personally, I feel that one of the great tragedies of the modern Western world is that we have forgotten or we ignore the real meaning and importance of the spirit. We claim to be at the peak of a civilisation but we really live in a barbaric age. Surely, if we were just a mind and a body, full stop, we would be nothing more than clever robots. Technology has provided us with machines that are capable of 'thinking and 'doing', but what makes a human being a unique and wonderful individual? What gives that essential quality and spark to human life: its experience of ultimate joy, understanding and compassion? The spirit – that is the spirit. But what importance do we attach to it today? I regret to say, hardly any at all.

Ignoring the spirit is the reason for not winning the fight against disease. We are abandoning and neglecting the deepest and most essential part of a person. If the spirit within us is denied, we will not keep in harmony and balance. Thus we will be more susceptible to disease."

The difficulty with defining what the spirit is, or what is also referred to as the "true self", is that it is beyond thought and words, and so paradoxically the key to understanding it (one of those Chinese contradictions) is accepting that you can't. It's a feeling thing and can only be understood through experience. It's apparent when you feel fully alive; the "goose bumps" moment when the hairs on your neck and arms lift and you feel something way beyond thought. There have been times in my life when nothing has touched me – everything feels very bland and functional – even things that in the past were so exciting. There's an enlivening feel about the spirit; sometimes small and quiet but exciting all the same, other times awesome and overwhelming but always indescribable in words.

The ancient Chinese had little problem in recognising and feeling the presence of "spirit" in everyday life. It was essential. This was a culture that knew from bitter experience that to ignore the spirit would be a threat to their own community and its long-term survival. They understood the "oneness" and interconnectedness of all life, and how spirit is the conduit between our inner and outer world. "As within – so without". For example, the warmth and fullness of summer mirrored by the open-hearted fun we enjoy at this time, and nature's activity in spring mirrored by the hopes and our plans we feel inside. This symbiotic relationship meant communication between the people and their environment was authentic and balanced and facilitated their success as a race. In our relatively safe and modernised world where our survival needs have changed, this natural attribute has been greatly diminished as our minds have taken on the impossible task of providing us with an authentic sense of self and a meaningful direction in life.

The breadth and potential of each human being's life is unfathomable to the human mind. For this reason, sadly, most of us who "think" our way through life only access a fraction of our potential, and for many different reasons limit ourselves to a relatively thin band of experience and suffer as a result. The purpose of acupuncture treatment is to balance our internal world so that we come from the right place - our authentic self - and to be at one with our external world. This harmonic, congruent relationship with our self and the world opens the door to the full life potential that nature and our spirit offers us, and in turn, we then contribute to the bigger picture of life in our own unique way. It's a beautiful relationship.

During acupuncture treatment this "tuning" is achieved by selecting specific acupuncture points that address the needs of each person, and it is through this provision that balance is attained. The "spirit" of all the acupuncture points combined tell the story and hold the mystery of life, and reflect the riches of nature and the world we see around us; the potential and capacity of each human experience is no less majestic than the whole of nature itself.

"Spirit Burial Ground", an acupuncture point located on the chest serves the purpose of resurrecting the spirit from under the weight of negative thoughts and experiences. On Geraldine it was electric. She woke up feeling hopeful and even happy for the first few days after her treatment, and we focussed on keeping her attention on the part of her that was healthy and well, lifting the old sense of dread for longer and longer periods. She realised for the first time that the love she had been looking for all her life was already present inside her. What we tried to do was to maintain that profound connection with her true self, her spirit, which had been neglected for most of her life.

At the Harley Street Clinic she was attending she did IUI, and after her third attempt she fell pregnant. She was at peace with the idea of being a single mum and I felt it was right for her to do this on her own at that time. Just a year after her baby was born, she met a fellow single parent at the park and is now enjoying a warm and loving relationship.

I had patient called Glen who was suffering from depression and had an extremely low sperm count. As we talked, he came back again and again to the idea that everything was pointless. He couldn't see anything succeeding so he didn't want to begin anything new. If he embarked on one course, he'd quickly find an obstacle and be knocked back to where he'd started.

He was unable to make a single decision. It was a longstanding joke among his friends that he would never spontaneously do anything. Even something as simple as the question of whether or not to take a bottle of wine to dinner foxed him. He drank too much and had previously had a heavy pot habit, and although he undoubtedly was talented as a choreographer, he didn't have the fight to try to create any new work, and was bumping along in a job he could manage without pushing himself. His girlfriend was despairing but at the same time accepted that this was "just the way he was", and hoped that a child would make a difference.

An acupuncture point located on the back called "Contracted Muscle" mirrors the moment when a taut bowstring is loosened. I used this point to help him release the pent up energy inside him, coupled with a point called "Spiritual Soul Gate" which, as the name suggests, gave him the capacity to experience his "spirit fly". The other main point I chose many times for him lay on the gall bladder meridian and is called "Great Mound", providing him a place of perspective to see beyond the obstacles he had created in his mind where he suddenly felt himself with a view and new prospects.

Before his treatment, I couldn't coax Glen to even begin to imagine what it would be like to be a father. It took some time to see a difference as his reflex to go straight back to that sunken depression was almost overwhelming, but gradually things changed and he became more sociable and even started going to the gym. He didn't stay for much further treatment after a doctor told him his sperm count had improved, so I don't know if they were successful in having a child, but things had certainly begun to shift for him.

Five-Element acupuncture is only one way to help balance the relationship between the body, mind and spirit, and from my clinical experience it is highly effective, but one of the most effective ways to maintain and strengthen this balance is to spend time in the natural world. Playing with animals and small children, listening to music; in fact anything that promotes a sense of peace will help, but most importantly be fully present in each experience in each given moment. Animals and children don't think too much, and if they do it looks quite painful. Watching my dog trying to understand my words is cute but you can see how much effort it takes. They exist in the moment, responding to life, as it happens, free to respond in any way that naturally arises in them – free and fluid.

Some of us are so far removed from the natural world and the blissful innocence of childhood that the only way we will reconnect with our spirit is to experience such a monumental crisis that our mind and body - no longer able to cope - quit! Numerous accounts of "spiritual crises" and the peace and contentment that emerge as a result demonstrate that the spirit is always there behind the thinking and the chaos. It's more a case of where we put our attention.

We focus on our minds and bodies by thinking and doing all the time, even when we go for a walk; we use this time to think rather than just enjoying being outside and walking.

Put simply – we are more than a body and a mind. The qualitative experience of being human comes from our spirit. We can listen to a piece of music with our physical ear, we can understand how it is composed with our mind, but the enjoyment and qualitative experience comes from our spirit. Fake flowers can look impressive and beautiful; we can see them with our physical eye, and understand that they look real with our mind. Our spirit however is not engaged. Body communicates with body, mind with mind, and spirit with spirit.

By putting your attention on your spirit, allowing your body and mind to rest, you start the process of aligning your body and mind *with* your spirit.

Balance – Optimising Your Fertility

Most guides to conception come with a list of do's and don'ts for what to eat and how to exercise from day one to day twenty-eight of the female textbook cycle, and a never ending list of don'ts for the boys. How much protein for breakfast, thirty minutes walk a day, sex when you ovulate, and absolutely no alcohol. For some people creating the right conditions to have a baby has become almost a full time job, or certainly takes up a huge amount of their waking day. The daily routines created by people trying to take control and doing everything in their power to conceive would be amusing if the implications of failure were not so high. Many people will do anything to have a baby, understandably, and if they read that it helps to stand on their head they'd do it.

Sally's morning begins at 7am with a pint of water, 20 vitamin pills and a piece of seaweed on wholemeal toast. Then off to a yoga class with just enough time to get to work at 9am. It's day 14 of her cycle and the ovulation test says 'yes' so she makes a quick phone call to John to check he will be home by 7pm (she read somewhere this is the best time for sex as her cervical mucous will be copious at this time!). She doesn't like her job and hasn't for over five years but the maternity benefits are great – so she stays. She pulls herself through the day snacking on nuts that stick in her teeth and annoy her, but a regular supply of protein is good for the blood (she heard that from someone last week).

Her partner, John, looks at his watch, puts away his phone and lights a cigarette. It's only one a day now but the guilt goes deep. He goes back to his desk and hears his colleagues laughing as they recount the adventures of the stag night he missed the Friday night before. His new life of abstinence, enforced relaxation and timed sex is taking its toll and he doesn't feel good.

And so it goes on for months and in many cases years. This daily routine is stressful and soul destroying, changing as each new tip of the week supersedes the last, rewriting the ever-changing formula on how to get pregnant. This process not only wears people down physically and emotionally but more importantly, spiritually. As faith and hope are slowly undermined by each failed attempt to get pregnant we dig ourselves into a desperate state that is both exhausting and depressing. People forget who they really are, and what they really like. Their relationships suffer dreadfully.

Very often these routines are so all-consuming that they enable people to entirely overlook the real underlying problems: that Sally hates her job – which she spends hours on every day – and John is consumed with guilt when he misses his old, fun life before he began trying to be a dad. And all the time, they're trying to fit themselves into a rigid way of life – their diet, their hours – which has nothing to do with them personally, and was dreamed up as a "one size fits all" cure for infertility.

Sometimes when I am treating people I ask them to do something specific like eating a decent breakfast or getting a certain amount of exercise, but it's by no means a militant approach. The most interesting thing for me as a practitioner is to encourage people to get a real sense of who they are and what works for them. Maybe they'd rather parasail once a week than go to the gym every day, or eat oysters simply because they enjoy it and it makes them happier than a zinc supplement. If you feel better for a night out, you feel better full stop. Guilt will hardly improve the situation or your health.

This isn't to say that a life of unthinking self-indulgence is the key to everything. The Five-Element approach requires you to step back from everything that is going on in your life and look again through the soft focus lens of your instinctive self. Without realising it, people have slowly slid into a way of living and a mode of thinking that seems normal to them but isn't remotely natural or good for them, and which could be negatively impacting on their fertility.

If someone is living completely out of whack, I recommend that they "reset" their system for three months using an approximation of what's called the Law of Midday-Midnight, or the Chinese Clock, which I will talk more about later. They may not carry every part of it on into their future lives, but some good habits will have been formed in that time, and most importantly they will have understood when and how they violate what Chinese medicine calls "the natural laws".

Violating Natural Laws

All of us violate natural laws every day of our lives. We ignore hunger when our stomach rumbles, eat when we are thirsty, take a painkiller for a headache when we know we should stop and rest, avoid confrontation when actually that might be a way of moving on in our life, and deny or delay an instinctive drive to start a family.

Some people are born with incredible innate resources that mean they can get away with pushing against the natural laws and against their health. Others might live just as long but have a weak constitution or live in difficult circumstances, and they constantly have to bring themselves back to that centre of premium function and to bolster that weakness through extra sleep, better food choices, healthy relationships and being more careful with their energy. You need to have a sense of your own limitations as an individual and not expect yourself to be able to cope with the same level of activities as others around you. You may be able to get by with less sleep than them, or you may need more. When you are in touch with your body and needs, you will be better able to judge this.

As we get older we often accept low-grade health as a norm. We feel "tired all the time" but don't connect it to not eating properly or exercising enough, or taking breaks from staring at a screen. We get used to being stressed and anxious as the little vices accumulate. We're like the frog in the pot of water, who does not realise that the heat is on underneath, and the temperature is gradually rising.

You wake up tired, so you kick-start yourself with caffeine before heading to a work environment that causes your cortisol levels to soar in response to the stress. You shovel down a sandwich at your desk and barely taste it. More coffee or tea to stave off that dip in the afternoon, and then by the time work is over you're cross-eyed and edgy, so of course you have an alcoholic drink to take the edge off. Too many drinks and you sleep badly, wake up tired and begin the cycle all over again. And of course it's all just "normal".

It's not that we're incapable of feeling as energised and relaxed in our later thirties and early forties as we were in our twenties, it's just that we lose our ability to judge that we are moving further and further out of balance.

Our body has already been designed with a perfect clock, so these good habits are latent in us, so to speak. The trouble is, our heads usually overrule it, and our lifestyles demand that we stretch it to the utmost. We think we can stay up all night and keep up our usual routine for the following week without any difficulty, and get surprised when we can't. The principle of homeostasis or a natural inclination to swing back into balance applies here too. You stay up till 4am one night, and a couple of days later you will pass out on the sofa at 8pm. Unless we try to override nature with coffee or caffeine drinks, nature will override us.

As much as nature wants us to procreate, its primary aim is for us to simply survive, so it won't put us at risk with reproduction in a stressful environment. Instead it husbands resources and shortchanges your reproductive capacity so that the rest of your body can cope with the harsh environment. Many men who present at the clinic with low sperm counts are in high-stress jobs, and are so set in their ways that quitting or coming off that adrenalin is unthinkable to them. Not surprisingly, their bodies are channeling resources away from their reproductive systems. Equally it is not uncommon for a women's menstrual cycle to stop completely when the pressure of life is on.

The idea that stress affects fertility has now begun to be considered by Western medics too. In May 2011, a scientific journal called Fertility and Sterility published the results of an experiment by Dr Alice D Domar, a doctor who specialised in helping patients to deal with the trauma of infertility. She studied 100 women who were taking a course of IVF treatment, 50 of whom were also following a "stress management" programme which included cognitive behavioural therapy, learning relaxation techniques and participation in support groups. After the second cycle of IVF, 52 per cent of the women who were being helped and supported conceived, compared to 20 per cent of those who had had no stress-management sessions.

Many major US fertility clinics now offer similar support schemes. Dr Domar told the New York Times, "It's not that it's all in your mind. If you're really stressed out the body seems to sense that it's not a good time to get pregnant." This is exactly what I would tell my own patients, although it can be hard to get them to realise that they are seriously stressed. Quite often when I ask people about their day-to-day lives, they don't spot the contradictions till they go through each part bit by bit – a chain of cause and effect quite different to what drove them in the first place.

I have one client who works as a stage manager in a large, busy theatre which means that she only works during the evening. This wouldn't be a problem in itself if she stabilised the rest of her time, but she wakes at eleven or twelve when she insists that she's not hungry, so keeps topped up on juice and hot drinks until five when she goes to the theatre for the evening. The atmosphere backstage is frenetic and she's at the centre of it all, instructing stagehands and making sure that actors and props are waiting at the right entrances. She still hasn't eaten anything by the time she gets at home at midnight, when she makes herself cozy with a book, music she loves and a big dinner, and sits up till 2am, whereupon she goes to bed with a full stomach and sleeps badly, only to begin the cycle all over again.

I've suggested that she maybe eats a proper breakfast when she gets up, meets a friend for lunch and has a light snack after the theatre and before bed, but she insists that it would be cruel to deprive her of this sacrosanct comfort zone. She's had the same habit for more than twenty years now, and has persuaded her body that it's not hungry for 22 of 24 hours of the day, setting in train an odd cycle of deprivation and indulgence. I think she would stand a better chance of having the baby she says she wants if she stopped overruling her appetite and paid attention to her body, but she also loves the life she already has, and of course she would not be able to keep the same schedule if she had that baby.

There is a point where nature will not allow us to continue pushing ourselves in this way, usually in the form of physical or emotional symptoms or even a spiritual crisis that tells us we have to stop and look at what is going on in our life and with our health. We need to understand that this symptom is an opportunity that offers us the chance to step back and change something, whether it's diet, exercise or a preparedness to be more honest with ourselves.

One woman I treated was head of a major multinational in the UK. She'd conceived three years ago, at a time when she was travelling back and forth between London and New York on a regular basis for frequent business meetings. She got off a plane one day and miscarried. She conceived again, and the same thing happened. Shortly after that she split with her partner and found herself in a very happy new relationship in relatively little time. They were both keen to start having children quickly as she was nearing forty, and worried that they wouldn't have much time.

They also bought a new house in the countryside, which, although pleasant and peaceful, was hours outside London. She started getting up early in the morning and kicking off work at 6am with her Blackberry and laptop on the train, which she thought was great. She then worked a full day in London and left the office at 7 or 8pm at night. On top of this, she still travelled transatlantically on a frequent basis and shuttled back and forth to Frankfurt, where the company was setting up a new office. She had a huge amount on her plate already when she came for her first appointment.

She wasn't an overtly aggressive person, but there was something jarring to me to the considerable energy that she gave off in the treatment room, as though she was constantly frustrated and wanted me to get on with things. She enjoyed her job and thrived on what she called the stress of it, and in many ways she had the reserves to deal with it, but perhaps not to hold a pregnancy at the same time as nailing down a major deal. It was as if her body had not even acknowledged her pregnancies when they happened – she'd felt no fatigue or morning sickness, but simply ploughed on.

The initial consultation and treatment had an immediate effect. I asked her to try to leave work at 5.30pm every day, and that she always took an hour out of the office to do something purely for herself; she chose a Pilates session at a local gym. I never suggested she should change jobs, but after a few weeks she jumped ship after ten years at the multi-national and walked straight into a high-powered job with a competitor. She and her partner had given up on conceiving naturally and were looking into travelling abroad to find an egg donor, and she was excited at the thought. Between the old job and the new she had three months of fallow period to make the transition, and it was during this that to her surprise, she fell naturally pregnant. This time round she experienced the full quota of pregnancy symptoms; she was tired and sick and hungry and needed to give herself time off to relax.

It was as though she surrendered to the physical changes for once, instead of letting her head overrule her body and cram in another meeting or two past 5.30pm.

She could have easily gone on with her busy lifestyle but in her individual case, something had to give. There are always going to be people who are physically hardy enough to conceive on such a regime and even thrive on it, even if they're not in their twenties anymore. But if you are trying to conceive, and run into problems, particularly those "unexplained" ones, a change of environment for that pregnancy might yield faster results than you'd imagine.

One case that my colleague, Anna, dealt with always appeals to me as a clear-cut example of ignoring the natural laws. Her patient was a young woman, only in her mid twenties, who was having no luck conceiving. She had a job cleaning tube trains at the end of the line at Edgware, where she worked a permanent night shift. She had one or two days off a week, but otherwise she was always asleep whenever the sun was up. Anna asked her how anything could grow without sunlight, and the young woman, taking the hint, switched to a day job and started walking out in the fresh air whenever she could. Within two months she was pregnant.

These stories confirmed to me once again that almost any of us are capable of returning to full health given the right treatment and support. It reinforces my belief and optimism that almost anything is possible when nature is given the chance to do what it is designed to do and we surrender ourselves to its plan.

The Law of Midday-Midnight / The Chinese Clock

Nature has a plan for you! The "Owner's Manual" was conveniently installed inside you when we were born and provides all the information you need to live a healthy, productive life and to survive in your given environment. This is great news for you - providing you remember to refer to it. Sadly most of us do not - not because of apathy or an impatience to get on with life but largely because we're not aware it even exists, and even if we know of its whereabouts we prefer to fumble through without it. I, like many people, used to hate instructions, so buying a new electrical appliance or anything that required direction was only going to have a successful outcome if pressing the "START" button was enough.

We typically take the healthy functioning of our bodies and minds for granted until something goes wrong. When we discover we're unable to make a baby it feels like our body has betrayed us, and yet many of us have been putting our bodies and minds under huge strain for years. Even the people who have technically been looking after themselves more often than not have been abusing their systems without realising it.

I recently visited a friend who was complaining about a plant he had bought from a local shop. "What a rip off", he moaned. "Fifty pounds for a brown stick!" he complained, and pointed to the skeletal remains of a Ficus Tree sitting in his window. I could see the small white plastic label that came with the plant poking out between the brown, crinkly leaves sitting on the dry soil. "You shouldn't place it in direct sunlight!" I helpfully commented as I read the brightly lit label.

Nature has designed us in such a way that every part of us will function at its best when we are in synch with our environment which is location and time sensitive. Our environment is always in a state of change and responds to the rhythms of day and night. The Law of Midday-Midnight is a body, mind and spirit "clock", that runs for a twenty-four hour cycle, broken down into 12 two-hour periods. In each of these two-hour periods, each one of your 10 organs and 2 functions that relate to one of the five elements benefits from an increased supply of energy – the peak flow. This two-hour period becomes their high point and a window of opportunity for them to function at their optimum. At this time they are most active and consequently function at their best. Conversely the organs or functions at the opposite side of the clock have less energy, and experience their low point, a time to rest, and are less efficient at their task.

I explained in an earlier chapter how imbalances in the five elements are frequently dismissed as personality traits; so too can disturbances in the Chinese Clock give rise to problematic symptoms and inappropriate behavior. For example many people say that they are not "morning people" and accept that half of the working day is written off. Others slump mid afternoon calling it a "carb crash" and collapse at their desk, and some who are stuck to the sofa at 7pm believe that an evening in front of the TV is all they can manage. On a glamorous night at the Opera, who wants to wait in line for the "loo for a poo"? Who relishes waking as bright as a button at 3am knowing there's a full day of work ahead? All these symptoms tell us our "clock" is running out of synch.

The law of midday - midnight teaches us the importance of "rest and play" and for us to respect the enormous and complex tasks the organs and functions do for us daily to ensure our general health, our reproductive health, and our survival. By ignoring this law we put extra pressure on these "Officials" and our system as a whole, and undermine ourselves as a result. The importance of the "team effort" is again emphasised here as any disturbance at any one period of the "clock" will immediately have a knock-on effect through the rest of the twenty-four hour cycle. When you work with nature's time schedule all areas of your health including your fertility are greatly improved and your whole system runs in one rhythm like a well-oiled machine. The following description of the Chinese Clock provides an understanding of how our organs and functions work and rest internally, and tells us how, ideally, we should live our lives externally.

The "clock" is a cycle and so we could start our journey at any point, but the early stirrings of a new day is a good place to begin. Between 3am and 7am, the metal element predominates and the lungs and colon are prioritised. For the first two hours your lungs benefit from the cycle's surge of increased energy, enlarging their capacity, awakening and oxygenating every cell in your body and every corner of your mind.

From 5am to 7am the peak flow shifts to the colon and has its best function – the optimal time to rise, have a bowel movement and release the physical and mental waste of the previous day. You'll remember the metal element is responsible for maintaining the "quality" of your health, and is achieved by the taking in of fresh air and the release of all waste.

Mavis Jones came to me almost 20 years ago, and at that time was in her mid 40's. Her main complaint was long-term infertility and chronic arthritis in all her major joints. I treated her at the first session and asked her to drink two pints of water every day. She was resistant to the suggestion, claiming that throughout her life she had never drunk water as she had grown up in a remote part of India where they only drunk tea and gin! She left, however, saying that she would comply with my request. Two weeks later she arrived at my treatment room looking radiant but concerned. "What have you done to me?" she asked. Reluctantly she started to describe the events of the previous 10 days; how three days after drinking the allotted water she woke at dawn, which was unusual for her, and was compelled to get up, put on her dressing gown and slippers and walk into her garden to sniff the air. It was autumn and the mornings were particularly frosty and unwelcoming. Immediately after this new ritual she would experience severe cramping in her lower abdomen and then sit on the toilet where "all this disgusting stuff" would come out of her. On further questioning it became apparent that it had been normal for her to have a bowel movement only every 10 days and that this daily excretion was new and quite shocking. Within a month her arthritis had completely gone away and she had her first menstrual bleed in 5 years.

Nature always gives before it takes. When a child clings to something it should not have, trying to take it away with force creates resistance. Distract the child with the offer of something new and the little treasure will hand over the original object with ease. We can see this in the case of metal and all the elements. When the lung opens and expands to receive the fresh morning air, this relative excess to the colon provides the release to let go. Nature ordains that all waste be removed at this time, and so in good health we empty our bowels, and shower away the waste from our outer lung - our skin.

Not surprisingly, the stomach is king over the next two hours, as the energy moves out of colon and surges into the earth element stimulating hunger and providing the energy to digest almost anything. The old saying that you should breakfast like a king and dine like a pauper is apposite. It's very basic – "nature abhors a vacuum" - and as you empty the lower part of your digestive system you refill from the top. You need enough fuel for the day. Would you really set off on a long car journey with no fuel in the tank? Fully satiated, the next stage from 9am to 11am is when the spleen is handed the energy baton and swings into action - transforming your intake into something usable for both physical and mental consumption and transporting it to every part of you to give the resources to move every muscle and get good thinking and working done.

The heart imbued with its daily energy charge rules from 11am to 1pm at the height of the day when it is good to relax and begin socialising - perhaps work meetings, conversation and joining friends for lunch. The small intestine then steps in to filter and organise from 1pm to 3pm, sorting and clearing the day's new information from things to keep and things to throwaway so you can have a productive afternoon of work.

Water takes centre stage in late afternoon and early evening between three and seven. First the bladder stores and reserves what you will later need. In western medicine it's just a sack for urine, but in the Chinese system it has the task of making sure you have enough energy for every task – a reservoir. It keeps reserves of fluid throughout your body, for your joints, your digestive system, your sexual excretions and tears. Lots of people experience a dip of energy in later afternoon because their reserves are low, but it should, if you are living by the clock and drinking enough water, be a time when you're feeling an abundance of stored up energy. The kidneys benefit at 5pm, when the body and mind's reserves are consolidated and you have a heightened experience of your own existence, and a profound sense of your "essential self".

At 7pm the fire element receives its second surge of energy as it enters into the two fire functions for the next four hours. It's a time for the circulation-sex function to come to the fore, a time for relaxation, socialising and sex, and being with other people rather than sitting at home alone. Interestingly this time period is the resting period of the stomach when this organ has the least energy available and yet most of us have our biggest meal of the day at this time. Is it any wonder our sex lives suffer? The second stage is ruled by the "three heater" or the body's heating engineer, busily traveling around every part of our being adjusting and correcting the physical and emotional temperature. It brings you down from the heat and activity of the day to a cool, resting state ready for deep restorative sleep.

The hour of sleep before midnight is important to start the natural rhythm of sleep. It is said, "an hour before midnight is worth two thereafter". Wood covers this hour and the three after midnight, when first the gallbladder takes the authority to redirect the essential inner activity of regeneration as you sleep, and then from 1am to 3am the liver steps up to store and detoxify the blood. It presides over the deepest sleep and the dreams that help your unconscious make good plans for the next day without the interference of everyday life. "Let me sleep on it", we commonly say when needing time to reflect and access the "vision" of wood and the liver.

What I found charming about the law of midday-midnight when I first learned about it was that it made me feel as though I didn't have to be completely in charge of everything. It also made me realise that there is an enormous intelligence at play keeping me alive while I am running around living what I call "my life".

In the West we're told we have the choice and freedom to work everything out for ourselves, and sometimes that freedom promotes an arrogance that is counterproductive. In the Chinese Clock your body and organs already know how they will best function, and how to give you the full life experience. If we work with them and follow the "natural laws", it all falls into place, and it's less of a struggle. Notice that the Chinese Clock has nothing to say about eating salmon or jogging for thirty minutes a day. There's room for flexibility, but you just have to acknowledge that by not working with this "law" you're not doing yourself any favours when the stakes are high for your health and fertility.

Any opportunity like this to find humility and be grateful for natural laws and our proper place in the world is a step in the right direction when it comes to conception - a simple moment in nature's work. The human mind is a relatively new phenomenon in the history of our universe, which of course means it is less well equipped to compete with the ancient law of midday-midnight. Obviously if you consistently violate natural laws without thinking or compensating for that swing out of kilter, then you will find that your body, mind and spirit will adjust. We are hugely resourceful, but it puts a huge strain on the system and eventually unease manifests itself in griping health problems, tiredness, gloom or unhappiness. Being fertile is a fine balance of many factors and nature records this balance moment by moment so as to only initiate conception when the conditions are just right.

Many of the people who seek help do so feeling well but are living in a false reality as the time bomb of ill health has yet to be revealed. Early warning signals are sent well in advance by nature, sometimes as early as 10 or 15 years; the niggling symptoms we get used to, a colour in our face we put down to fatigue, a spate of restless nights we blame on noise, unexplained infertility we cannot understand.

Men Vs. Women

The World Health Organisation figures for global fertility are as follows:

- One in six couples are infertile. In 40 per cent of cases the problem lies exclusively with the male, in 40 percent with the female, 10 per cent with both partners and in a further 10 percent of cases the cause is unknown.

- One in 25 males has a low sperm count and one in 35 is sterile.

There are huge variations all over the world in these numbers, but this breakdown still shows that infertility is a shared problem between men and women.

I have tried to include as many examples of men as possible, because as is clear from statistics that infertility can affect men and women equally. If there are less stories centering on men in this book, it's not because they play a lesser role, but simply because they are generally more reluctant to seek help and I have worked with fewer men by far.

Twenty-three years ago when I started working as a psychotherapist my clients were mainly women and gay men. When I qualified as an acupuncturist the same two groups made up the vast majority of my patients. As I began to get a reputation as a fertility specialist, there were even more women in my practice, even though in many cases it was the male half of a couple who needed treatment, and not the female.

We live in a culture where for thousands of years women have been given sole responsibility for conceiving (or not conceiving) babies, and that notion still dominates. There are far more fertility procedures which deal with women's bodies than those of men, who are often given a clean bill of health after just one good sperm test. It's women who congregate at web communities to discuss menstrual cycles and diets, commiserating and bonding, and not men, whose feelings on their own infertility are often far more private, though still deeply felt.

The majority of women who come to me still turn up on their own, and continue to have treatment solo. It can be difficult to persuade men to involve themselves because they're often more cynical about alternative treatments like acupuncture, psychotherapy, and in general seeking help, and they also look at how the money is being spent on supplements and IVF with few results. If the doctor has said there's nothing wrong with their sperm, they don't see why they need to change anything about their lifestyle. I see men taking their responsibilities as fathers seriously the moment their child is born, but it's rare to see a guy who's on a special diet and working out in order to further improve the quality of his sperm and his chances of conception. Generally their attitude is that if their female partner wants to pursue an alternative route of help, she should go ahead, but not drag him into what he sees as women's business. When their partner then turns round and says it would be a good idea for them to have some kind of treatment, they normally resist.

If one half of a couple makes changes to their life – be it through therapy, acupuncture, a change in diet or any self improvement class – it's often the case that they suddenly make a leap forward and in some way create a greater separation from their partner, who then seems left behind and stuck in their existing way of living. I try to encourage both men and women to prevent this kind of thing happening – asking for help and making changes isn't just about getting pregnant, but about improving your quality of life. It seems a shame that only one half of the equation should benefit. Times have begun to change though, and I've seen a steady increase in the number of men seeking help for all kinds of problems and not just infertility.

A good example of how men can get lost in the system is evidenced in Michael's story. He originally came to me for a chronic toothache that had been going on for years and only responded for brief periods when treated with antibiotics. He was in his mid thirties, worked in television and lived in South London with his girlfriend Janet and her two sausage dogs – Samson and Delilah. During our first meeting he was absolutely tickled that I was asking him about his childhood when all he wanted was localised pain relief for his tooth. When I moved on to do the physical exam and felt his spine and other areas of his body, he burst into hysterical laughter. "This is mental", he spluttered.

People find it very strange that we take so much time to take a full medical and personal history before addressing any symptom. This however is a good example of a situation where a long-term chronic condition like toothache can have a much deeper root, often missed in Western medicine by only focussing on the presenting symptom. If the body is not responding to medication there must be some underlying cause that could also be affecting other areas of his general health. Michael casually mentioned that he and Janet had been trying for a baby for over three years. I asked him if they had had any medical tests for fertility and started to explore what was wrong. Seeing my confusion with what he was telling me, he then confessed that although his sperm results were excellent, he had erectile problems, coupled with severe and very painful eczema around his genitals to the extent that they rarely had sex and were now considering IVF as a way of bypassing these problems. His acceptance of the situation was courageous in some ways but there was also something rather sad and pathetic in how a serious condition was simply swept under the carpet because of the availability of medical interventions like IVF. What would have happened prior to the advent of IVF? So, poor Michael now has antibiotics for his tooth, IVF for his impotence, steroid creams for his eczema – what next I wonder?

Who's Having the Baby?

As a couple get caught up in the system it is easy to move further from the original core meaning of conception, of a passionate coming together of male and female, as one or the other falls by the wayside. It's usually women who seem fired up to take responsibility for the process, although I have seen the same happen with some men. They have the enthusiasm for the new diet, or the new treatment, or this thing they heard which worked for so-and-so. The other half is soon a passenger, feeling increasingly ambivalent about the whole thing. As a lot of men shy away from the medical world even when they don't have a clear problem, they are easily left behind in an unfamiliar world of blood tests and laboratories and appointments with professionals.

Those men who do plunge in often do it out of a sense of duty to their spouses, and they don't seem to have that same desperate drive as women. Sometimes buried deep down are very private feelings about the whole process. Men have to contend with a lot of built-in notions of pride and shame; that you're not a real man if you can't get your woman pregnant. They're supposed to be nonchalant about the process and sometimes are, to the extent that they get left behind and all but left out. Feeling sidelined by the course of events, it doesn't occur to them to keep themselves in shape in order to maintain the quality of healthy sperm. Often I'm shocked when a new male client tells me their age – it can be ten years younger than I would have guessed.

What sometimes makes this worse is the way in which women, being the first ones to seek help, make new professional relationships with a practitioner like me, or their gynaecologist or their fertility guru. Because they're talking about their deepest hopes and fears and the most intricate, secret physical and sometime emotional issues, they rationalise this openness by forming quite an intense and personal bond over this problem of conception, making it more of a project between the woman and the professional, and less between her and her partner.

Suddenly the fertility expert becomes teacher, best friend and magician all rolled into one. Women queue to get onto the waiting list for this or that doctor, about whom there's been so much discussion between their friends and on a fertility website they frequent. First it's "Dr" this and "Mr" that, and in no time they're on cosy first name terms. They throw all their hopes into this one individual and his or her team, making them into their new support system, and stop focussing on their partner and the relationship which should be the very core of their desire to have children. The man is expected to play his part by providing sex and sperm, and after that's over the woman reports back on progress to her real buddy in fertility – the practitioner.

Keeping partners of either sex involved is essential, with not just practical changes of diet or exercise, but also simple communication and affection.

Balance "With a Twist"

On Tony and Karen's first visit, it felt as if I was I was having a consultation with one person. Tony talked for Karen, in language that ran the two of them together. He'd say "When we were last pregnant", or enthuse about the textbook menstrual cycle "we" had had that month. They had been hoping for a child for over 5 years and in that time "they" had had 3 miscarriages in the year prior to seeing me. As we talked, I realised that the pregnancy had become very much Tony's project, almost to the exclusion of Karen at times, who seemed happy to let Tony take the reins. She was happy with her job, with Tony and her life, and if it turned out that they were unable to have kids, very unusually, I don't think she saw that as a disaster.

Tony, though, was clearly a very sweet loving man, but to my mind excessively involved in everyone else's lives and readily admitted his nickname was "mummy"! He wanted to look after everyone. He didn't really want to talk about what he did at work, he would rather share the ways he'd helped work colleagues and friends who'd come to him with a problem. There seemed to be something jarring in how he was behaving. He also proudly admitted that he wanted to stay at home with the new baby once it was born, rather than go to work.

He was genuinely a very caring man, and there is nothing wrong with the impulse to care for a baby, to look after people and to be a good friend, but with him it had become such an urgent and grasping need that it seemed to dominate the aspects of his personality which you might call traditionally masculine. I think too, that the flip side of that need to help friends was his need to be helped and supported by them, which had become a kind of projected action. More often than not it's a woman who can lose enthusiasm about her career when faced with the challenging issues of infertility and rely on her male partner to keep the show on the road while dealing with this problem.

I referred Karen to see one of my colleagues and began working with Tony myself. After a few months there were no great eureka moments, but a gradual sea change in the man. As he slowly started to recognise his own needs, his focus drew back a little from his friends and domestic life, and I found him taking on new hobbies and contracts at work with attack and enthusiasm. With his new salary he organised and booked a surprise holiday for himself and Karen, which made him immensely proud. Karen was essentially very well and hadn't needed much from treatment, and although neither of them had any diagnosed problems before treatment, it was only after that sea change and a romantic time away in the Maldives that she got pregnant.

I'm not for a minute saying that men don't make great househusbands, or that they should never be in touch with their more feminine side. Quite the opposite, as in Chinese medicine the correct balance of yin (female) and yang (male) in every person is the foundation of good health, and this book is essentially about balance. Women are predominantly female and men are predominantly male, but everyone is a blend of the two and this paired dynamic is witnessed in all of life. For example, we see it in the seasons, the silent power of winter moving into the rapid growth in spring and peaking with the full blossoming and heat of summer – considered the more dynamic, male side of the year. The more receptive and female side is witnessed in late summer, producing the harvest and drawing everything back down through the autumn to preserve life through the winter.

Through their observations of the natural world, the ancient Chinese paid particular attention to a dynamic that not only maintained their life but also created new life. They called this natural phenomenon the Law of Husband and Wife. This law states that in nature, and so in every person, immaterial of their sex, the husband side of the energy must slightly dominate the wife side in order to keep the wheel of life moving in a forward and creative motion. The Five Elements follow the order of the seasons, the life force flowing upwards on the husband side and flowing downwards on the wife side. The husband side comprises of water that creates the wood, wood that feeds the fire and fire that produces the earth. The wife side sees fire producing the earth, earth creating the metal, and metal giving form to the water. This is the natural order and so this law states that the husband side must always dominate the wife side.

This statement can make heckles rise in a modern context but we have to remember that when the Chinese were developing this system of medicine they lived at a time where the primary focus of life was one of survival and so each person played to their strengths.

Both the active and receptive forces we see in life are powerful in themselves and essential; don't get blinkered by the Western idea that the active role is somehow better than the receptive. There needs to be a qualitatively greater force on our husband side to initiate life and equally there needs to be qualitatively lesser force on our wife side to draw life back down and conserve. This is something that must exist in each person and will not necessarily be evident in the relationship itself. Interestingly we see this in the body – acupuncturists take the pulse of both wrists, and the left, or husband side, should always be qualitatively stronger.

What the law of Husband and Wife teaches us is that there is a natural balance of opposites found in nature and ourselves. We are all unique and some men are more feminine and some women are more masculine – this is normal. However, when there is a disturbance within the relationships of the five elements we can often start to see a disruption to the natural balance within that person and inappropriate behavior and physical pathologies can develop and appear to become part of the person's make-up. It is not a way to judge or support stereotypes of men and women but simply to recognise and support a part of the cycle when it is in distress.

This is a very sensitive area for discussion, particularly as the roles of men and women have changed dramatically in the West over the past 100 years. It is clearly evident that high-flying businesswomen and stay at home dads can conceive as easily as anyone else, providing these roles are authentic and rooted in a path that naturally unfolds for each person. Some patients I have worked with have taken jobs that are ill suited to their nature but they pursue their career to satisfy other's expectations, stereotypical roles, and to prove something to themselves. This choice comes at a cost, as going against our nature will inevitably produce symptoms of some kind to let us know we are taking the wrong path.

Tony did not fundamentally change from treatment – he remained a kind, sweet person, and there was certainly no chance of turning him into a red blooded alpha stud – why should he? The change that seemed to make the difference was that his care and concern over becoming a father became more appropriate and substantial, and rather than just talk and talk, he started the walk the walk with real integrity and then found success.

Relationships

I am often asked about the importance of "the relationship" when it comes to conception. Is it more likely to happen when we are engaged in a healthy, happy wholesome one, or does the story of a relationship make any difference at all? I really don't know - but what I have noticed over the years is that happy couples get pregnant, feuding partners get pregnant, single people get pregnant; equally these same groups don't get pregnant, and interestingly some practitioners working in the field of infertility have sidelined this issue by completely ignoring it. How often are you asked about the nature and health of your domestic life with regards to your fertility?

Relationships are wonderful and inevitable but they can also be messy, in fact quite ugly at times, and just as the weather will change outside your window, one moment calm, the next moment stormy, so will the dynamic between the people we see inside. It is simply not true that fertility is dependent on a Waltons-esque environment. Babies are conceived in all kinds of relationship varieties; loving and warm, cold and indifferent, bully and victim, some even as a result of rape sadly, so we must observe and accept this fact and look further for truth.

A notable and very interesting observation I have made over the years while treating patients, is that the people who have struggled to conceive and have then gone on to be successful, seem to be the ones who have significantly improved their relationship with their "self", and their general health - regardless of whether they are coupled up or not. Of course, being in a healthy relationship rather than an unhealthy one is important to our overall wellbeing, but a relationship itself does not seem to be essential when hoping to conceive. If pushed for an answer, I would say that authenticity is the key. Being in an unsatisfactory relationship is not a problem as long as you admit it to yourself and accept it for what it is. However, deluding yourself that you are living a fairy tale romance that doesn't actually deliver may have a negative impact on you, your health and your fertility.

Fertility comes increasingly under the microscope of western science and the already established "department" approach to health and healing dominates when looking at the causes of infertility. Is there a problem with the woman's reproductive organs? Is there a problem with the man's sperm? How are the hormone levels? How are the mechanics of the tubes? This approach to treating fertility is medically brilliant, but it is also segregated and a clinical evaluation of a situation, rather than inclusive. Because of the sheer stress of the process it can separate the often long-suffering couple even more and create or exacerbate any problems in the relationship. Along with all the stress and emotional difficulties of trying to make a baby there are also logistical issues that can get in the way and unless addressed and dealt with, many weeks or even years are wasted, thousands of pounds lost, not to mention the disappointment and further damage to the relationship as couples are firmly placed on the infertility conveyor belt.

A woman I treated when I first started practising came in for help with unexplained infertility as she was about to get married to her long-term boyfriend and wanted to have a baby as soon as she could. There was clearly an issue in the relationship, but I had only been treating her for three or four sessions when she surprised me by saying that she'd realised that she was on entirely the wrong track. I'd encouraged her to be honest with herself and me about her feelings, and to connect with what really felt right to her, and she had come to realise that not only was she with the wrong man, but the wrong sex of human altogether. She had always felt drawn to women, but had pushed away the instinct because it didn't fit into the pattern of life that was expected of her. She split from her boyfriend and almost immediately plunged into a relationship with a woman, had a child with donor sperm from a close friend, and has been so happy since that she counts her blessings and sends me a Rosh Hashanah card to say thank you every year. Two other gay women I treat who are using donor sperm have been told by the clinic they are attending that they are not allowed to get pregnant at the same time because they are in a committed relationship. This "now it's your turn" approach has caused all kinds of stress and competitiveness between them, especially as they are both in their early 40's and feel under an enormous time pressure.

There are a tremendous variety of people struggling with fertility issues, each with their own characters and individualities and quirks, and I've seen unlikely matches that worked and "ideal" relationships that turned out to be painful and complicated.

Mike and Francesca were the perfect couple. I met them together for the first session, and immediately found them very pleasant and impressively dressed. As we chatted, they took it in turns to lead the conversation. Having already agreed which of them would speak about what. They called each other dear and they had regular sex. They'd met at exactly the "right" time for their careers and had a lovely house in west London with its own gym, where they worked out side by side every morning before going to their workplaces where they were each on track for excellent careers in competitive industries. They had one "perfect" child, and wanted to have another, but for three years nothing had happened and, after a clean bill of reproductive health from their doctors they had come to see me. Why weren't they able to conceive again?

If anything disturbed the perfect impression they gave, it was an absence of something at the heart of the relationship. They were just neutral. Not angry, not happy, not sad. Their desire for a second child was the only exceptional thing about their emotions and even then, it was a very tidy sentiment.

When I saw Francesca for a treatment on her own, something else started to emerge. She was very dismissive of everything, worst of all herself. I'd ask her about what she'd done that week and she'd begin "I read this book the other day..." and then, out of the side of her mouth, add, "Tssch, like I read." This tic carried over into everything. It was almost as though she had an imaginary friend to whom she was saying what she really thought, and all of it was self-deprecating, and she was oblivious to how strange it was.

I didn't feel like I was getting anywhere with her for two or three months, when she suddenly let slip that every time she got her period she would be so disgusted that she would begin to hit and beat herself. The language she used when she told me was vicious, like a louder, more vituperative version of her acid asides about herself. This confession turned out to be her big breakthrough, and after that things began to accelerate in an extraordinary way.

The first thing that happened was that her previously clockwork menstrual cycle broke down, and suddenly she was having a period after three weeks, or after five weeks, and then three again and then nearly six. She was freaked out by the change, and it seemed to bring a trail of chaos into their well-ordered lives.

They started coming to appointments talking about arguments they'd had with each other, with their friends, with their parents, whom they'd confronted over something. When she told me what had happened that week, the stories were about arguments and fallings out, but they were now animated and full of life, and she had no time to add a self deprecating aside. She complained about Mike and the way he'd behaved on holiday. She was furious with her father over some dispute about money. Everything the couple had brushed under the carpet before now got an airing as they scrapped over their most crucial beliefs. Their

117

perfect façade was replaced with something more passionate and vital. The treatment they got at the clinic messed them up thoroughly, but it also brought them to life. That neutral emptiness gave way to all sorts of feelings and in the midst of all the chaos, Francesca finally conceived, to everyone's astonishment.

The pregnancy was difficult. Francesca had terrible morning sickness and needed to take a lot of time off work. At the same time Mike was promoted at his work and moved to a new office with a long commute from home. He would leave the house at 6am and rarely be home before 9pm. Francesca continued to struggle well into her second trimester until one morning she received an anonymous phone call from someone telling her that her husband was having an affair. Devastated, she called me for an appointment, arrived at the clinic and completely broke down. Rather than be angry with Mike she expressed complete disgust for herself, to such a point I really thought she might leave and take her own life. The intensity of her grief was profound and there was nothing I could do other than hold her hand as she descended into the deepest pit of self-loathing I have ever seen. Remarkably, very suddenly the sobbing stopped - she looked up at me and through bloodshot swollen eyes and smiled. It was over.

Francesca's sickness disappeared overnight and the rest of her pregnancy was as normal as anyone could expect. Mike apologised for his indiscretion and it seemed that through this enormous shake-up of their perfect life, they found a point of balance, having swung hand in hand from one extreme of the pendulum to the other.

I love a happy ending as much as anyone, but let's not be fooled by the romantic idyll of couples who find all the answers by simply forming a magical union; relationships take work. This story might suggest that by allowing the natural chaos of life to enter their artificially perfect world, a window of opportunity was opened for new life to begin. Maybe – but from my experience it is very important to not get too hung up on the quality of the relationship as an entity in itself, but to look at the individuals that make up that couple.

I have come to recognise that the enduring relationships with the real happy endings are the ones where each person takes complete responsibility for them self, independently of the relationship. Healthy relationships grow when the individuals each do whatever it takes to be well, regardless of the outcome. Mike and Francesca had obviously papered over their own personal cracks when they first met and were very pleased with the great joint result, until it fell apart.

Sometimes the social pressure driven by the "biological clock" theory makes people panic into relationships that they know in their hearts aren't right for them. I treated a woman called Molly who had found a nice boyfriend called Declan through Internet dating in her late thirties, and after months of dating happily and taking a holiday together to test the water, they decided to get married. They'd both specified in their online ads that they wanted to have children, and so they began trying after the wedding, but there were no results after a year.

When she saw me for the initial consultation she told me that she was depressed because she had been unable to conceive, but when I asked her about Declan, she'd just shrug and say he was fine, alright. They hadn't been together for that long but she didn't sound excited about the man – what he did, what he said, all those things that someone in love will tell you, unselfconsciously, ad nauseam when they're smitten.

Declan had moved into her flat, and after a while the basement flat directly below it came up for sale. She wanted to buy it and knock the two apartments together, but found that instead of reaching for this chance for a family home, Declan had simply given up his job and was quite happy on the sofa being supported by her. Had she become pregnant at this point, who knows what would have happened, but instead she just grew more miserable. I began to push her to see if she really cared so deeply for Declan that she could overcome this, and he really was the right person, but instead, after a lot of tears, she confessed she had rejected many partners along the way and had been holding out for the love of her life, and now at almost 40 even this one didn't make the grade. She ended the relationship and stopped treatment. I'd sensed before she left that it was deep down a relief for her to escape this sanctioned partnership that she'd tried to force to work, as the world was telling her, but the knowledge that it would take her longer to have a child hurt her more than the loss of Declan.

Ending a relationship when you know time is running out can be one of the most painful of all experiences and the agony is not only because the chances of becoming a parent have just decreased, but also because we insist on believing the cultural myth that someone else is meant to make us happy. In Molly's case the rude awakening was a blessing in disguise as she could easily have become completely comatose and compromised her own values and the dream most certainly would have turned into a nightmare. Our culture pumps out constant messages that support this flawed idea that we need a relationship and that someone else who will bring us love. What we fail to recognise is that we are the only ones that can make us feel truly complete.

One couple I saw had had one child and were trying for a second, but where the wife made every effort to appear warm and full of life and love, her husband would sit next to her and contradict and criticise every second thing she said. He was sarcastic and made demeaning jokes which she simply laughed off. The contrast between the two of them was marked. They had been through nine rounds of IVF and technically there was no reason why they should not have another child, but he lost interest in acupuncture after a few sessions and there was little change with her, as she had, I think, chosen to maintain her own fantasy about what she described as a "wonderful" relationship. The dynamic between them was so inert and cold that if conception needs energy and warmth I couldn't imagine them being successful again.

As much as we enjoy believing someone else will bring us love, no one out there is capable of loving you as much as you love your self, so the starting point for all relationships begins at home in you. You loving yourself really means that the generation of love happens within you – it is a self sustaining dynamic not dependent on anything outside of you. It is also worth remembering the Taoist philosophy that teaches us the law of cause and effect; there is a cause, and you and your life are the effect! Relationships with other humans are the effect of how we feel about ourselves. What we love in other people tells what we would like for our self, and what we deplore in others is inevitably something negative lurking in us.

When we are wishing to have children and it doesn't happen, we want to do all we can to get the picture right and create the best environment. Yes, a good relationship can be part of that picture, but a relationship with someone else, outside of our self is just a romantic story. If "relationship" does enhance fertility, it's worth remembering that your greatest and most potent relationship is the one you have with your self.

Bigger Relationships

Healthy human beings enjoy other human beings. We are sentient, sociable, loving creatures blessed with an enormous emotional capacity to love and to be loved.

The majority of us no longer live in a society where the extended family provides "in-house" security, love and support. Families are often spread over many miles, even continents, and have little or no contact with each other. In the face of childlessness a common response is to see it as a secret problem, conceal the issue and engage with our will to try and find a way to make conception a reality, a desperate need to find and correct the problem and get what we want, a baby and a future.

A young couple, Peter and Judy came to me at the end of their fifth year of trying for a child. They were both very stressed and exhausted, having just completed their seventh round of IVF. Every attempt had failed and they were desperate. The most incredible part of their story was that in the five years of hoping to become parents they had not told anyone else about the gruelling process they were going through. Judy worked as a graphic artist and Peter worked for a television news channel. They were both in their mid 30s and had regular contact with their families and appeared to have a wide social network.

They seemed perplexed that I was so surprised at their need for privacy. When I asked how it felt to keep such a secret, they became defensive and told me clearly that it was a personal issue and "no-one's business!" I was curious and pursued my questioning by asking what they told people who asked them if they planned to have children. Judy's rehearsed response was, "No, we don't like children; we are more interested in our careers".

I felt this shroud of secrecy around the issue was intense, almost shocking and had become habitual. When Judy was doing IVF she had to visit the clinic daily for blood tests and would tell her work colleagues she was doing a course to learn a new computer programme. When they were invited to parties where they knew children would be, including their own nephews and nieces, they would intentionally avoid them in an effort to support the story that they had no interest in becoming parents.

It was painful to hear how thwarted their life had become. On the surface they were two successful people in a loving relationship and had everything they could dream of, but underneath they were broken and desperate, bound by their lies and living in the shadow of their secret.

"I don't want sympathy!" Judy barked at me as I suggested it might be helpful to share with someone. "No-one understands. All of my siblings have children. How could they help with our situation?" Judy had all the answers. Unconsciously or even consciously she was trying to exert control over a situation where she had no control. She apparently knew exactly how her family, friends and work colleagues would react if they knew. "They would be embarrassed and not know what to say, so why bother?"

It may have been true that the anticipated response

would have been exactly as she expected but what Judy and Peter seemed not to realise was that in five short years they had moved from an open, honest relationship with the people around them to a closed and dishonest one that was causing a great deal of pain.

When I suggested this could possibly be part of the problem they were, understandably, not convinced. They had heard that acupuncture could help increase fertility and so they wanted needles and results, not whacky suggestions. I treated Judy for almost two months and in that time there were some improvements in her health and general well-being but there was still something in the way, evident in her constant underlying anxiety and almost pathological fear of family gatherings.

Infertility can be a lonely journey. Often the responses of other people are unsympathetic or tactless: one client who was undergoing IVF for a second child had just had over twenty embryos transferred into her uterus without any of them implanting. When she was told by a stranger that she was wrong not to have had a second child because "only children are a lot of what's wrong with this world", she looked at her healthy, happy son and wondered what this stranger could possibly hate about him.

Given these negative responses, it is not surprising that fertility problems are often kept a secret from others; some people carry a deep sense of worthlessness and shame. It's usually a result of ignorance as much as insensitivity, which is a symptom of the same problem. The truth is we are here together, trying to get along with each other and share human experience. Our sense of separation from each other is something we choose. In reality we are totally dependent and interdependent on each other.

Secrets are hidden inside us, tucked away from others, often concealed and given little room to breathe. Secrets can be hidden because they are of great value and must be preserved, or because they are shameful and painful. For the most part they simply need the light of day. 'A problem shared is a problem halved', and if we can find the right person to share our secret or problem, the simple relaying of the information can be enough to effect a significant change in us. It didn't help Judy to tell me her 'secret'. I was a professional person who would support her through this time but it meant nothing to her for me to know what she was going through.

Much to my amazement Judy came to a session one day and told me that she had finally announced to her whole family the truth of their 'unexplained infertility'. She now felt like a different person and her family turned out to be supportive in a way that she had never imagined possible. When I questioned her on why she told them she simply said that she had no choice, she needed their help; the words had just suddenly come out.

Judy and Peter re-engaged with their families and in particular the nephews and nieces in a way that had felt impossible before, but now that the "strategy" was in shreds, they were free to get on with life and enjoy what was on offer to them. During an extended summer holiday spent with Peter's brother, wife and two young children Judy conceived naturally and now has her own two little girls.

Being around people is good for us. Being open and honest about both our failures and our triumphs is healthy and normal and gives us the kind of freedom we witness in nature. There is day and there is night, sometimes things go well and sometimes not so well. This is the normal healthy balance that nature teaches us. We can also learn a lot from the experiences of others. One patient, Polly, spoke of her relief when she found another mum at the playgroup who had had difficulty conceiving a second child. Another, Martin, said it was great to talk to friends who had adopted children when he and his wife were considering what to do next.

Asking for help takes humility and courage, but the very act of asking requires great strength and has the power to change a stifled and stuck situation. Sometimes we forget to ask; we make the decision that we want something and we employ our will and set about getting it. However, the simple act of asking with all your heart to be given what is right for you is enough, and your right action will follow. It is gentle and easy and usually works. Some call it prayer, but whatever name you wish to give it, don't forget to ask.

Sometimes being open isn't so much about trying to conceive, but rather to reveal underlying tension. I met a young woman who was fairly newly married and had been trying to get pregnant for eighteen months. Yet again, she was a case of "unexplained infertility".

Neither she nor her husband had any health problems and they were still in their twenties. I asked her why she thought she couldn't conceive and she said she had no idea.

I began to treat her and we chatted during the consultation about her life and how she felt. She mentioned that she had problems with her in-laws, which her husband wasn't sympathetic to. This seemed like a common enough problem, but when I found out a little more I discovered why it was disturbing her so much.

She was white and her husband was black, and although his family had been perfectly sweet to her, she was struck with a sense of hostility emanating from them. She tried to talk to her husband about it, but he didn't think his family were at all racist and said she was just being paranoid. The in-laws were very polite and said that the couple were welcome to stay at their home, but she couldn't face it. "There was something about the way the wedding was organised," she told me, "as though they were trying to keep people separate."

When her mother-in-law phoned and talked to the husband, he would barely be off the phone when she would ask him if his mother had asked about her, and they rowed frequently about it. He felt that she was rejecting his family for no reason, and she was haunted by the idea that not only did her in-laws secretly resent her, but that her husband too didn't really love her. She wanted to be with him, but her instincts were telling her that she wasn't welcome within his family and that she was pushing him away by being so distraught.

I found her so wrought up that I suggested one day that she openly asked them if they had a problem with her. The next time I saw her, she told me she'd gritted her teeth and gone to his parents, proud black British people, and they'd assured her that no, they had no problem with her at all.

Now the tension really began to build up. Her husband was angry that she'd effectively accused his parents of racism; his family were rattled by her claim. In the end it all came to a head when she was talking with her sister in law who broke the family silence and admitted that yes, it was true, the family had been uncomfortable with having a white daughter-in-law.

For a while there were accusations and hurt feelings thick in the air as everyone finally came clean. Her husband was nonplussed. Her in-laws were embarrassed now that their true, racist feelings had been revealed. Then, suddenly the storm cleared and everyone was strangely relieved that the big secret was out in the open. Instead of the family splitting at the seams and estranging the young couple, or their relationship collapsing under the strain, they set out wobbly into a new future as a family. Two months on, she conceived her first child.

We like to believe that we know what is going on around us. We think that people only know what we choose to tell them and we limit our understanding of others to what they have chosen to tell us. It keeps life simple and safe, but on the odd occasion when people are brave enough to challenge us on perhaps what they see as our insensitivity to them, we defensively shoot back, "but you should have told me". The truth is that we are communicating on many conscious and unconscious levels and collecting enormous amounts of verbal and non-verbal information all the time. In fact, the majority of information that comes out of our mouths is so flawed and inconsistent that we would be better to shut up completely if we really want to be understood.

These two stories of where honest, open, loving communication transformed lurking tension and menace and possibly opened the path to conception, remind us of the intelligence of the natural world. New life is born out of appropriate conditions dictated by natural laws. A code of deceit and manipulation and the stress that combination produces in the body is no different than soil that has been polluted by toxic chemicals - highly unlikely to foster the germination of a seed.

Love

Love is a frequency. We are just like a radio receiver that can receive energy and turn it into sound, and a transmitter that can produce sound and send it as energy. Love has its own vibration and is rooted in what I have been describing as spirit. We cannot experience love in our heads, and as brilliant as the human mind is, it is simply not designed to tune in. The mind works at the level of thought rooted in the physical, and is there to interpret our experience but is not the experience itself. It is really important to understand this and to recognise the difference; otherwise we get ourselves into all kinds of confusion.

For the ancient Chinese, it was simple; "love" was life itself. The gift of this planet, the rising of the sun, the seasons changing, even one's own existence: everything natural was a state of love. Love was seen as the active part of life that powered evolution and was benevolent in every way. The creation in spring and the destruction in autumn - the essential balance of these two seasons that turned each year and maintained life – was seen as loving. When we observe nature, we see the creative cycle of the elements and how each element is created from the unconditional love-thrust of the previous element, the original mother/child relationship. By observing how nature creates a cycle that is so absolutely loving, giving and effortlessly flowing, we understand what occurs within us - not because of us, but despite us.

Love is about acceptance and humility. The acceptance of ourselves, the laws of nature, the situation we find ourselves, our friends, our lovers or partners and our children. If we accept others as they are and take full responsibility for how we feel about them, regardless of what they do, say or believe, we enter into a loving state, which takes maturity and is healing and life enhancing.

On the other hand, the comparatively unseasoned states of "falling in love" and "falling pregnant" are involuntary acts that can catch us off guard at any time. So, is love a trick of nature to keep the species going? Is love itself an active ingredient in making babies? Are we more fertile when we are in love? Are we disadvantaged if we are trying to conceive and love is not in the picture? Within our current medical approach to fertility "love" certainly does not figure at all. Conception is largely seen as a biological phenomenon that sits apart from any emotional influence.

So why do we fall in love? and having "fallen", why is it that we resurface as the honeymoon phase comes to an end? The generally accepted explanation of what happens when we fall in love is that we return to a very innocent and natural state. This was around the time that we were born and shortly after, when we were almost pure consciousness. With our sense organs only just beginning to develop our only real experience is that we were "at one" with everything. We merged into everything around us – we had no boundaries. We couldn't differentiate ourselves from our cot, our mother's arms, our location; we were simply an ecstatic bundle of energy and form. In this precognitive state, providing we were given what we needed, our response to the world was spontaneous and completely unselfconscious.

As we developed we became aware that everything and everyone was separate in the world of form. This included our newfound thoughts and labels that named our separation. We realised that everything has a name - we have a name; that we have two arms and a head and that our parents are separate entities from us. What came with this discovery was the loss of that original experience of being fully integrated with everything, a sense of Oneness. Our love of babies and the reason that humans enjoy being with them is that their innocence, their newness and fragile state, taps into something we love and remember, our non-material self; our spirit. When we fall in love the self created ego cracks, our boundaries are loosed and we experience a return to pure being and love; no judgments, no preferences – our existence is eternal and blissful.

When we are in this trance like state, every part of us functions at its optimum, including our fertility. Falling in love fast tracks you to a place where everything seems possible and is the perfect state for self-abandonment and conception, not to mention the bonus of a greater frequency of sexual activity.

If you are no longer "in love", be assured that this fall from grace is completely normal as the honeymoon period wanes. This relatively brief window of experiencing the blissful Oneness of life feels like a tease of nature for us to blend and merge. Being in love is a relatively artificial and temporary state, that changes our perceptions, and can feel like the experience of taking drugs that take you up and take you down. How many of us didn't notice our lover's annoying habits when floating on cloud nine; he slightly hunches when he walks and she doesn't shave her legs. As the ego boundaries click back into place, so come the judgments; the critical mind to re-establish separation, and the inevitable question – where did my soul mate go? At this point hopefully, the "mature" adult steps in, whose heart and mind finds compromise, and accepts the other person for who they are, and embraces every part of them with an acceptable and sustainable love.

My patient Anna was a great teacher for me. At our first meeting her physical beauty and her strong presence immediately filled the small treatment room and for a few moments I was completely thrown. When she spoke she locked eyes with me and lacked any self-consciousness as she told me she wanted to have a baby but needed to find a partner first. In the next breath she asked me if I was married. I smiled nervously and chose to change the subject by asking another question; she looked at me suspiciously and folded her arms. Her bold and intimidating style was seductive but it also felt aggressive to me and I was starting to lose control.

The nature of rapport between the practitioner and patient is crucial to success in diagnosis and treatment. The relationship is professional but is also dependent on a certain openness and transparency which must be managed by the practitioner. This fine balance can be hard to achieve, particularly when the patient has the skills to cut through the professional veneer. Anna was a master and the first patient to really wobble me. I already felt on the back foot and I could feel myself scrabbling to find my ground. "Why won't you tell me if you are married?" she asked. "It's a simple question". I finally gave in and confessed that I was single, but that wasn't enough. "Why?' she asked defiantly. This precocious "child" was not giving up, but I managed to find my way back to centre and conduct the rest of the consultation drawing on, at that time over 15 years of professional experience, but if she was out to test me, she was good.

Anna told me she was depressed. She was 36, had a very successful career in public relations and was adored by a string of men who would do anything for her but she said hadn't found "the one". When she described these platonic relationships, she was effusive and generous in her praise of these men and reeled off the holidays and gifts they continuously bought for her, but it seemed strange to me that none of these "wonderful" men had made the grade, and that they persisted, surely knowing that they were never going to get what they wanted. Two of them had been "courting" her for over 10 years. There was something that Anna was doing that kept them all dangling.

As our sessions together continued I started to feel a disconcerting push/pull dynamic between us, never feeling I could get it quite right with her and needing to remind myself that I was not her lover and did not have to feel responsible for her happiness – but I did. This was troubling for me but also a very interesting challenge as I had to presume that whatever she was managing to induce in me was the same as all the other men in her life. I never knew how she would be with me; sometimes sweet and affectionate - speaking in a tiny girly voice - and at other times cold and shrill, making completely unreasonable demands. She tested every boundary I created, pushing me and seeing if she could cross it; she knew my weak spot and would go for it like a shark to blood. After four sessions she asked me again why I was single. Rightly or wrongly I told her I was a "confirmed bachelor". "So, are you looking for someone?" she shot back at me. This whole interaction was shocking to me on so many levels, my head was spinning with personal affront, professional confusion and panic on how to return serve. I paused, said nothing and the moment passed.

After she left I couldn't help wondering if she had found the perfect challenge in me. Unavailable as a partner, unavailable as a lover; Anna wasn't just having trouble with self-love and finding a partner, she now wanted a partner that wasn't allowed. By inappropriately going after what she couldn't have, it's possible that this was a way of denying herself the chance of having a child. It became clear over many months that Anna struggled with any kind of adult emotional intimacy. She was childlike in her demands and expectations and it became clear that no one would ever be able to give her what she felt she needed.

She said she felt "unloved" and alone and yet it sounded like she knew half of London and had possibly the most feverish social life that any one person could handle. She was unable to benefit from all the love around her and she was so distrustful of her relationships that she was caught in a love/hate dynamic with everyone. Just when I thought I had totally upset her and would never see her again, she would return with flowers and a card with the most elaborate loving sentiments. It was painful to see how she struggled, how hard she worked to manage these countless relationships with people and ultimately, how none of them gave her what she needed.

Anna is a great example of someone who possibly either didn't get the love she needed as a child or was given no boundaries, but more importantly she didn't know how to generate love for herself. She simply couldn't be alone, always on the phone, always planning the next visit to someone, somewhere. She also believed that once she found the right man and had children of her own she would feel complete. This is part of that western myth that deludes so many of us. As I said before, there is no guarantee that anything out there will ever truly bring you love and peace.

Anna stopped having treatment when I confessed after many months without much progress, and with great relief, that I wasn't sure how I could help her. Working with her had brought up many issues for me as a practitioner. She came to me to find a partner and get pregnant, and even though I try my best not to collude with patients' desires, it was very hard to keep the focus on where I felt Anna was really struggling.

She was a kind, loving and generous person whose spirit shone so brightly you couldn't help but be completely mesmerised by her, but she had to find a way to be self-sustaining and generate love for herself. It is tempting to believe that it's someone else's responsibility to bring us love, and some people manage to maintain relationships where that is the case, but how much better to create and enjoy love for our self, and then share with everyone we meet.

Love is the universal mix, the great creator and binder of all life and is present and available to us at all times. If we are unloving, or feel unloved then either we have lost our connection with the source, or we took the misguided step of thinking we could do it alone. The ancient Chinese had a sophisticated and allegorical understanding of how love manifests in humans. The "utmost source" - an acupuncture point on the heart meridian - receives the source of love, the "mandate of heaven". This raw essence of heavenly lore is then transformed by our own little love factory, the circulation/sex function, to generate unconditional love for ourself and others.

What this ancient wisdom teaches us is that we as individuals are the creators of love in our life; we are love. Just as our western culture has spun us the myth about relationships, so too it tells us that love and happiness are to be found outside of our self. We are lead to believe that we are damaged if we were unloved by our parents, tragic and pitied if we never find a loving mate, and useless and lonely if we fail to have kids. The stakes are high when we buy into this myth which produces all kinds of neurotic behaviour that can only be described as madness when we look at the lengths we will go to chase this illusive love and joy. For those of us who have had enough, we reluctantly turn our back on love and call it a day.

Despite all of Anna's difficulties and internal conflicts, two years after we abandoned working together she returned to me with an acute case of morning sickness. She had accepted a marriage proposal from one of her more ardent suitors the previous year and was now four months pregnant.

Do I believe that love will facilitate conception? Yes, absolutely, but it is not necessarily the romantic love you might have been expecting.

Sex

In talking about love and relationships, it's impossible not to bring in the question of physical passion. When people start out in relationships they have sex in what you might call a normal fashion – in other words, when they feel like it. They want one another, they want to see the physical response of the partnership they're building, and they generate a huge amount of passion.

Lots of couples now leave years between meeting and settling down and finally having babies. When they have difficulty conceiving, it's often the (unspoken) case that their sex life has settled into something comfortable and comforting and a little routine. Often when couples set up their campaign for conception they mark out a timetable for sex in this or that margin around this or that fertile period. Later along the fertility conveyer belt, they have started scheduling sex for strict periods of time around the woman's ovulation, using graph paper and thermometers to stimulate sex rather than, say, a sudden, sexy inspiration. It strips all that primitive energy from straightforwardly fancying someone and doing something about it on the spot.

You don't just lose lust and pleasure, but also intimacy. You stop having sex if it's not the designated period. Little by little the whole process is dehumanised, and the relationship is undermined. I often first see people when they've been on one of these regimens for two or three years, and they're so focussed on having a baby that they haven't even noticed what's happened, and assume that as soon as the woman conceives their old love life will just slip back into place without a hitch.

It's easy for all of us to forget the mysterious and exciting time of our pubescent sexual awakening, the innocence of child play eclipsed by the rising serpent within, transforming us and our perception of our playmates into sexual beings and objects of desire. The freshness of this time carries a vital potency that is hard to maintain beyond our teenage years and early 20's, particularly if our sexual activity is focussed around one partner. The dynamism of this early sexual arousal carries the energetic charge designed by nature to ensure the survival of our species; desire more often than not overwhelming rational thought.

This exciting time, however, in many young people's lives is overshadowed and blighted by the ever-present "fear" of getting pregnant as Anita explains:

"I don't think I'm alone in having a complete fear and horror of getting pregnant drummed into me throughout my teenage years. A pregnancy would ruin my entire existence, stop me from completing my education, ruin my parents' reputation, drive me to a backstreet abortionist and possible death – it really was the worst thing that could happen. Consequently, many of my generation thought that rabid sperm lurked everywhere, just waiting to catch us unawares and get us pregnant – we all knew that it only took one!

So I went on the pill, used Dutch caps, condoms and coils, determined not to be part of the tragic teenage mum statistic, and tried to dissociate sex from procreation. But I always thought that without these magical safeguards I would be pregnant in minutes.

Years passed and I found myself at thirty wanting a baby. I had also gathered the husband, the house and all the trappings that were required to provide for the anticipated bundle of joy, and thought that all I needed to do was stop taking the pill and bingo! That's not exactly the way it played out. My four years of unexplained infertility left me feeling a complete and utter failure, at times suicidal, worthless, bitter, twisted and angry with the world. I couldn't understand why something I had tried so hard to avoid (like a disease) was now eluding me, and why everyone else – and people without my advantages – could apparently do it easily.

The self-loathing I was filled with every time my period started was horrible and must have been equally miserable for my husband. I lost all interest in sex unless it was the right time of the month while feeling the whole time my husband should leave me and find a "proper" woman and that all my other achievements counted for nothing. I was incapable of seeing any joy in my life that wasn't associated with getting pregnant".

When you have had this kind of experience it is hard to find spontaneous desire and passion when your mind has already been primed to house negative messages around sex. Every experience we have in life is recorded by the mind and immediately turned into memory. Memory, much like old photos that remind us of something in the past, cannot hold the spirit and freshness of the present moment. So when we engage in sexual activity, often only because it is the right time of the month, and with the same person in the same bed in the same way, even though the event is fresh and new, our mind can trump the experience by playing out a memory, dull and void of life. The mind is so powerful that our partner could transform completely before our eyes and we would barely notice the change as the old tape keeps playing in our mind of what we think we already know.

Our desire for the freshness of the new and the trick of the mind to keep us in the story of the past is often the cause of sadness and frustration leading to affairs and sexually compulsive behaviour, and rarely has anything to do with a problem in the relationship itself. Thinking and sex are as compatible as oil and water. Fantasy, like role play, is not of the mind but is creative and spontaneous; so the real trick to bringing back the love into our love life is to get out of our heads and back to our senses where everything is new.

We adults think far too much. I've sat in the treatment room and listened to people have telling me that they've heard that mobile telephone signals will go through their bed springs and stop them conceiving, so they've decided to have a bed made with no springs. Someone else told me that she wouldn't let her husband wear brown because it deadens your energy and she'd bought him a magnetic bracelet to boost his sperm. I've had clients who have studied so much that they could go head to head with Sir Robert Winston on Mastermind about fertility drugs or the benefits of an all-cabbage diet on pre-menopausal women.

However, if I ask patients how their love life is, they're shocked and stumped for answers. Suddenly they've run out of theories and graphs. When I suggest that a couple overhaul their sex life with perhaps a romantic weekend away, some role play, maybe some toys, or really anything that gets them in the mood, they're even more shocked. They protest that they're too busy and tired for that, but if they're too tired to have sex I have no idea how they'll cope with a baby. They blame their in-laws – they come to stay too often – or themselves, "It's my fault, I don't always feel like it," anything to push away that awkward challenge. When men have erectile problems, the process gets pathologised and there's a prescription for Viagra: it becomes a condition to be medicated, not a temporary blip in a grand passion.

People would rather open up their folders and bring out their charts and tell me all the homework they're putting in – special diets, charted ovulation, correct positions – than go away, rethink, and have a heady holiday of sex for the sake of sex. I hear all about cervical mucus quality or the number of sperm in each ejaculation, but to mention the bedroom gets them bristling – in the wrong way. Perhaps if I came out with a statistic to say they would increase their chances of conception by 60 per cent, they would do it. It is very odd to sit with couples who intend to be together for the rest of their lives and raise a family, and watch them make excuses for not making love or finding real sexual expression.

Having sex is just a grown up version of playing,

and the child inside us misses the games. Unlike the dead memory we sometimes evoke during intercourse games are fresh and alive. Sex is meant to be playful and joyful and provides an arena for fun, experimentation, fantasy, intimacy and loving expression.

First person: Sally

"If you're lucky, there's a feeling that you get sometimes when making love with someone you are completely passionate about. You feel so joined to him that you almost become him; your body is so open and receptive that it feels as if your womb is unlocking and taking him to your darkest, most primal secret places. I would say this is the prime conception shag! And if you add a bit of desperation into the mix, it can get even more heady."

The self-consciousness that comes with age and ageing can extinguish the flame of passion and in many cases of the couples that I have worked with, non-verbal agreements are made to take the easier option of a cosy cuddle and a peck on the cheek at night.

There are good physiological reasons found in conventional scientific research for concentrating on the quality of your sex life instead of your ovulation schedule. One study in Australia found that the more frequently men ejaculated, the higher their sperm quality. IVF clinics had been telling men to raise their sperm count through abstinence, but the researchers discovered that although this resulted in more sperm, much of this multitude was made up by a backlog of old or even damaged sperm which was not improved for being kept stewing! On the contrary, the men who ejaculated on a regular basis had a smaller, but far healthier population of fresh swimmers.

In any case, sperm quality can vary hugely from week to week or even from day to day, as I will explain in more detail later. This variation is another reason why we recommend that people trying to have children have sex every other day – it's pointless having sex only a few times a month when the woman is ovulating in the hope that the man's contribution on those particular days will be up to scratch. By ensuring a fresh ejaculate of sperm enters the woman's body every other day you increase the odds that there will be at least one champion to reach the egg. Sperm can live from a few hours to anything up to five or even seven days inside the female body, so it makes sense to be sexually active at least seven days before the expected ovulation and a further three days after. But procreation is not an exact science. Having regular sex, amongst other things, sends a clear message to the body and mind of both the male and female that there is the possibility of conception. The human being is intelligent on all levels and understands what is going on and will respond accordingly.

As for women, regular sex actually stimulates ovulation. Women with active love lives release an ovum in ninety per cent of their cycles, compared to women who abstain, and whose egg release drops to less than fifty per cent of cycles. Nature doesn't squander its resources if there appears to be little chance of the egg being fertilised!

Not every woman ovulates at the same stage of her cycle – it depends on the health and state of mind of a person from month to month, so it's often impossible to calculate ahead when sex is most likely to "pay off". This problem is avoided if you are having sex regularly and for its own sake.

Even Taoist philosophy recognises the significance of our sexual union, signalling the end of "separation" and taking us back "home". Our instinctive drive to couple up, build sexual chemistry and climax is not simply to produce new life, but to reconnect with something far more exciting than anything our body or mind could generate or conjure up. Symbolically, the merging of heaven and earth and the end of separation is expressed through the sexual union of the predominantly male (heaven) and the predominantly female (earth) - where two become one.

Practising acupuncture in the Taoist tradition, and witnessing the success stories of many patients who resurrected their sex lives and went on to conceive, I have no doubt that the magic of conscious, alive and connected sex improves your chances of conceiving enormously. Male and female, yin and yang, merge and the resulting physical, mental and spiritual union nourishes every part of us and reminds us of both our humanity and our spirituality; our sexuality.

As much as we are persuaded to believe that conception is a purely biological phenomenon, I have no doubt that there is something beyond our understanding at play when new life emerges from the dark. Conception is still a mystery as is evident in the low success rates of IVF. When on paper there seems to be no reason why the procedures don't always work, it's still a lottery. Human passion and the feeling of being alive cannot be ignored when looking at conception. We are not inert machines performing dry functions trapped in time and space. We are vibrant, energetic beings with a limitless energy source if we only knew how to harness it. Do you remember how much energy you had when you fell in love, or found a passion for a new project? Where did that come from? This life giving energy is available to us at all times and one of the most fun and exciting ways to access it is through sexual expression. Being sexual and loving is very human and adds an extra dimension to our life that brings energy and light to everything we do, and very possibly could be the missing link in the "unexplained infertility" chain.

The Importance of Orgasms

Did you know that if a woman has an orgasm either a minute before or up to three minutes after her partner, her body will hold on to ten million more sperm than if she came long before or after him or even hasn't climaxed at all?

The actual mechanism of the female orgasm is so intricate and influential that new things about it are being discovered every year. Why else would women be able to orgasm if it served no purpose other than pleasure? Pleasure is only one side effect of the sequence of events set in motion by a climax; the rest can make the critical difference between conceiving and not conceiving if a couple are having difficulties. There's even a chance that ovulation can be triggered by surges of hormones pre- or post-orgasm, or, more incredibly still, that the contractions of the uterus in climax might shake the follicles into erupting. Orgasms also have a bearing on how the woman's body treats the sperm that's ejaculated.

The vagina is naturally acidic and hostile to sperm, even containing roving phagocyte cells which will consume invaders – all part of the vagina's self-protection system. Most sperm perishes there and then, although the vagina's pH is briefly raised so they can survive a short time. If sperm is lucky, it finds a way into the safe haven of the cervical mucus, which has reached lower down the vagina with the cervix, which also dips down as the woman is stimulated. The contractions of vagina and womb create higher pressure in both. When the woman climaxes, the pressure in the uterus drops sharply, and the cervical mucus and the sperm are effectively sucked up through the cervix and drawn closer to their ultimate destination; the ovum in the fallopian tubes. Also with male orgasm there is a greater volume of sperm ejaculated when the period of arousal is extended. Taking time to stimulate each other will increase the power and potency of the orgasm as a whole.

In short, it's more likely to happen when you're highly sexually aroused, unthinking and surrendered. Again and again patients have confided that they got pregnant that time they had amazing sex on holiday, or went on top for the first time. There's a real excitement and dynamism, like Sally's "prime conception shag".

I've had male patients who gave up up their old partying lifestyles to go to the gym and sit home with decaf coffee, and I've told them just to go out with the boys and have fun. No, you can't conceive if you're overdoing the party lifestyle, but to exclude that abandon and fun and flirtation from your life altogether is too extreme. Often people are simply bored and worse still, scared, convinced that if they get smashed on tequila they risk having damaged babies with this or that abnormality. The most extreme example I ever witnessed was a woman who had been unable to conceive for years despite her partner having no fertility problems, but who got pregnant as the result of an impromptu wild sexual encounter; freed from all her anxieties and issues by a quantity of champagne, she slept with two men and now has a gorgeous daughter to show for that extraordinary evening. I'm not recommending orgies for everyone, but there must have been sparks flying that night!

One pair of couples I know in the USA had no problem conceiving twice even though in this case they were two gay men and two gay women. Each couple made love in their own rooms, and then the sperm that the men had gathered was passed over to the women (who both happened to be doctors), to apply after their own orgasms. Their children were born out of making love and of an orgasm that was fuelled by love, even if the biological mothers and fathers were in separate rooms at the time. When I talk about what is natural and of male and female coming together, it doesn't have to strictly mean a single heterosexual couple: that energy is generated from love and passion.

I do also believe that a sexy, passionate session can improve your chances of a successful implantation if you have undergone IVF or ICSI or a similar, clinic-based procedure. I suggest to patients who are about to have an "embryo transfer" that they should have sex before they go for their appointment, because the heat and chemical reactions of orgasm prime the womb to receive a new inhabitant. Otherwise the new cells are simply transferred from a cold, sterile laboratory environment to a relatively inert uterus, instead of a post-orgasmic one that's pulsing with blood and receptive. I also suggest to people undergoing assisted fertility treatment that they maintain a sex life throughout the whole process leading up to embryo transfer; even though technically it is not needed, I am guessing that those who manage this regular sex have a higher chance of success than those who are simply focussed on their blood results.

A certain erotic dynamism can change your whole body make up, making you a more vibrant, sexual being. When you flirt with others – even with no consequences – your body responds. If you look at teenagers, they're still excited about getting out to socialise, to meet people and make an impression. It may look like spending hours on their wardrobe choices, but in fact it's honest excitement. When couples find one another and settle down in their nice, comfortable house, they often take this to mean that they can retire from the social scene to some extent, and that lack of interaction makes them less sexual beings over all.

I am very aware that frequent sex isn't practicable for everyone. You can choose to go to the gym or take a walk each day, but you can't compel your partner to have sex with you. In those cases, there's possibly another underlying problem with the relationship, or one or both partners is being dragged down by emotional baggage that I will talk more about later. I find that when two people are feeling better in their skin and healthier inside and out, the knock-on effect of that tends to be that they feel sexier and more attractive. They're more excited, they have more energy, and that spills over into an increased libido and a natural spontaneous desire to make love.

Love, sex, relationships and orgasms are all essentially the same thing manifesting in many different ways. The starting point is always love - the juice of life - and in many spiritual traditions "love" is

considered the only thing that is real and lasting–
everything else comes and goes.

A Balanced Mind

The ancient Chinese teach us that "spirit" is perfect and always present; it doesn't need resurrecting and it doesn't go anywhere. It's us that come and go, but sometimes it feels like our spirit has been completely buried by everything that has gone on in our life. By the time you hit your mid-thirties you're mentally a composite of many influences from your DNA to your parents' relationship, your peers at school, messages in the media and your life experiences. As we grow and respond to the world around us we develop an idea of who we are and what we believe to be true. This construct gives us a personal viewpoint and a framework from which we live our lives, but if we are not open to reviewing these ideas and actions they can equally become a trap and restrict our movement through life. They're like bad mental habits that we don't even recognise as holding us back.

Over years of practice I've learned that most of what people tell you in a consultation isn't the full truth. It's not that they intentionally lie, but the past is a story that can be changed in the present and frequently is, as we all need to find reasons for things we don't understand. If you treat patients according to what they tell you, you have to trust that they're right, but usually they are telling you nothing more than stories. Patients tell me that their terrible backache is because they fell out of a tree 35 years ago, or that they can't sleep because their house is on a ley line, or that their terrible indigestion is just like their mother's or their aunt's. Yes, it's true that women do have a genetic predisposition for certain things like, for example, their menstrual cycle and menopause, but there's normally something more going on when people seek to line themselves up with their parents or anyone else to explain their traits, or worse still come up with theories based on hearsay. We take things from our experiences and turn them into a story we tell about ourselves; we say we are impatient because our mother always made us wait for treats, or that we have a bad stomach because that's just how it is for all the men in our family. We think we're night owls because we can't sleep, or we have bad blood sugar and that's why we need to binge occasionally. We reckon that we love the adrenalin of stress, or that we're just one of those people who gets sluggish and hibernates in winter.

I often ask patients how they feel right now, rather than collect past history, and if, as so often, the answer is "exhausted" or "depressed" or "stuck", my next question is to ask them why they don't change what they're doing and so change how they feel.

Recently I saw a new client who had been trying to get pregnant for five years. Doctors had discovered that she had a breast tumour three years before she came to the clinic, and after an operation she had been given an all-clear. I asked her what had been going on in her life in the years immediately before this diagnosis, and the first thing she burst out with was that her parents had an almost derelict house in Cornwall, and that they'd stuffed it with bric-a-brac from antique shops. "They don't know how to look after themselves," she said, then "I don't want to live like that." It seemed an odd thing to say as of course no one was telling her that she had to.

She went on to say that in order to keep her parents' house under control, she'd been travelling from London to Cornwall every second weekend to check up on them and sort through the new bits and bobs they'd bought. She said they needed help organising it all, or else they'd be overwhelmed in no time. "Do your parents want your help?" I asked her, "Oh no," she replied, "They like the mess." "Why do you do it then? Isn't it a lot of hassle making the trip every two weeks?" "I do it because I can't stand the mess," she insisted.

That's when it dawned on her that her weekend drives to Cornwall weren't about her parents after all, but about herself. She was trying to save them from the thing she most feared; that if she had no children there would be no one to look after her in her old age. She compensated for this with overbearing behaviour towards her parents, who were quite happy with their lives. She made herself the carer, the "only one" who worried about the things that needed to be worried about, but she was doing this for people who were only humouring her and didn't require her help.

She worried, she said, all the time. She was sure her partner didn't really understand her, so, I imagined she subconsciously was wondering how he could look after her in the future. My job was to help her move out of this state, and so the first thing to do was to break the habit of displacing those concerns onto her parents, and not head off to Cornwall to tidy their house for at least six months. She needed to accept that her partner maybe didn't have a perfect understanding of her – few people do – and to stop worrying about that and understand herself and enjoy who she was instead.

She had a fundamental insecurity in herself, and had been expecting others to step in to fill that breach. This possibly had a knock-on effect on her fertility, as who knows if her body was prepared to bring a baby into this scary environment that she'd created for herself. I strongly felt that if she was able to create her own sense of security and feel safe in herself and be self reliant, she would be able to conceive.

When people like this new client present themselves a certain way – in her case as the worrier and the carer – they have gone far beyond seeing their behaviour and all the associated feelings as an imbalance or something inappropriate. They define it as their personality. Of course, having one of the five elements as their causative factor will produce a tendency to one emotional direction, but I've also seen that temporary swing off the scale corrected by a combination of acupuncture and self-willed change by the patient so quickly that it belies the idea that it was ever an ingrained part of who they really are.

Another patient, Julian, was an actor and son of a well-known artist. He'd been in therapy for years without making any progress, and had a diagnosis of depression, although he came to me for help with his fertility because he and his wife wanted to start a family and he'd been told that he had a very low sperm count. As I walked round the treatment table to take his pulses, his eyes followed my every step. It struck me that the atmosphere in the room was not one of depression – a dragging, sunken greyness – but instead of high tension and anxiety. He could only articulate it as "a black feeling".

Fear is often not given its due. People talk and write articles about depression and the devastating effect it can have, but how many men can admit to feeling afraid, let alone take time off work for anxiety? It is not recognised as something that could be so chronic as to be an illness, and yet I see it cripple people over and again. When Julian described his working week, it was clear that what drove him was a wild surplus of adrenaline and anxiety, and not soul-sapping depression.

Julian said he could never settle. He worked most of the time at home writing screenplays and occasionally did some acting work in the West End. At home he would pace around the room, his mind darting and coming up with thoughts too numerous to write down, and then he'd open a bottle of wine. It seemed to me that both these tactics were a way of trying to burn out and then dowse the fear. Only when he was too exhausted to do anything else, could he finally sit down to work. After that, he was good for nothing of an evening. The anxiety wasn't removed, but just run ragged until he was in a state of extreme fatigue.

After he had had treatment over several weeks he started to show results. One week he went away and returned for his next appointment saying in surprise that he'd felt a difference; this time he actually called it "an absence of fear". He seemed refreshed and less manic, and said he'd drunk less alcohol because he hadn't needed to cope with "the black feeling". Next time he came back, he had swung back into extreme anxiety but this time he recognised it for what it was, simply a passing feeling. I continued treating him and gradually that swing back to "normal" stabilised, and he was both able to work more easily and to father a child when his sperm count recovered significantly.

He eventually told me his earliest memory of that black feeling. When he was a child his father would force him into his studio and sit him down at his side. The boy would be given paper and a pen and told to write stories as his father worked. They would sit together in silence for hours at a time, the little boy forcing himself not to fidget and to fight the urge to run about and play. It imbued him with a terrible feeling that, as a seven year old he couldn't place, and that grew worse when his father would ask to hand over the pieces of paper and let him read the story or essay he'd written. No wonder as an adult he couldn't bear to tie himself to a desk all day after years of silent fear and sitting in that studio.

No one exists in a fixed state. You don't need to remain scared forever because of a childhood experience. Many of my patients describe aspects of their lives that sound absolutely miserable and yet they battle on as though they cannot possibly escape their situation. They have lost a sense of perspective. They hate their job but feel unable to change it. They don't like where they live but they'll come out with a reel of reasons for staying there. Julian thought he had to drink to write and almost saddled himself with a serious alcohol problem in the process, without seeking out the source of the emotion that drove him to be so scared and restless.

Many years ago I was treating a woman called Charlotte who was 32 and had been doing everything possible to conceive for almost three years. There was nothing wrong with her medically and she said she'd had a happy, stable upbringing and continued to enjoy her adult life. She called her life "picture-book perfect". She and her husband had been very successful in business and she felt secure and loved by him. The only thing missing was a baby.

Not long after starting treatment her father was diagnosed with lung cancer and told he had three months to live. He also told Charlotte that he had excluded her from his will because he thought she was financially stable and well off through her own endeavours, and wouldn't need further support from him. Her brother had very little money and was assured a significant figure by their father, and her sister would get the balance. They were all a little mortified by their father's announcement, and had promised Charlotte that after his death they would share out the inheritance equally, but the damage was done. Charlotte felt rejected and as though her own father thought she was worthless.

She thought her idyllic life had fallen apart over night, and she sank into a very dark place full of self-loathing and fear. I worked with her to support her through this sudden depression and early grief, and she did her best to understand why this had been such a blow. This involved taking a close look at the story she'd told herself about both her upbringing and her current life.

When she was little, her father was a god. She was devoted to him, and described the moment when he walked in the door in the evening as "like the sun coming out from behind a cloud". Her father was devoted to her too, and would take her everywhere with him, but one afternoon when she was twelve he took her out with him and introduced her to a female friend he called Jane. The three of them spent the day together but Charlotte felt very uncomfortable with this woman, and noticed, even though she was young, how close her father seemed to her. She never did find out if her father was having an affair with Jane but from then on she felt that the special relationship she'd had with her father changed irrevocably.

When her father told her about the will she was pitched back to this time when she'd seen her father through different eyes and been disappointed in him, and left feeling alone. She hadn't realised at twelve how deeply she'd been hurt, or that she'd felt betrayed. Rather than talk about her feelings with anyone, she'd tried to cut her father out of her affections without thinking. That emotional separation marked her. From that day on she'd gradually come to see everything as her responsibility, and her drive had been to create and control a perfect life that couldn't be shaken by someone else's betrayal. The woman I met at the first consultation was strong, charismatic and determined to

161

create and defend this life, and her father had obviously understood that she needed nothing for him. He in turn had felt rejected, although at a conscious level all he had seen was success and independence. His last will and testament reflected this unspoken deal.

When she stepped back and saw this chain of events, Charlotte saw the pattern of emotions underlying them, and talked to her father and found herself ready to forgive him. She shifted gears in her own life too – she began to enjoy the comfortable life she had created for herself without striving to defend it or submit it to anyone's approval.

Her father defied his diagnosis and lived a full year. Charlotte was with him the night before he died and felt no resentment or anger, but only love. She conceived her first child exactly 3 months later to the night.

Another client, Robert, had been told that he had an incredibly low sperm count – literally forty or fifty in a sample. He was only twenty-nine and newly in love with an incredibly sweet woman with whom he wanted to have children. They hadn't been trying long before they went for tests, only to be brought up short by this dire result.

When I put my hand on his chest to check his temperature, it almost felt as if his whole body was going to suck me down and keep me there – he loved the physical contact, any form of contact. This was obviously a deep need for him, and yet even with this tremendously kind affectionate girlfriend right there with him, he was still desperate for any affection. It was as though he couldn't produce this feeling for himself and so always needed to absorb that care from others.

He also wanted to help others, telling me his plans for learning to be a hypnotherapist and putting together a package of ways to assist people in losing weight. He'd done all his research and knew there was a good market out there, but you could see what it really meant to him – an opportunity to care for others.

I asked about his medical history and he told me that as a nineteen-year-old he had been recruited by a fast-growing technology company that prized his brains and put him onto a fast track for promotion. He was full of ideas and fresh perspectives on the business, and his bosses began to portray him as the company superstar who was destined for great things. He worked hard, pushing himself to meet their expectations, but at twenty-one he was completely burnt out and suffered a nervous breakdown.

He collapsed and left work, battling depression and paranoia at home. He was given antidepressants and counselling, and managed to get disability benefits. He was out of the work place for years, living in much reduced circumstances, and the psychosomatic symptoms that he suffered could be crippling. He felt dizzy constantly, and his stomach lining was gnawed by ulcers. Slowly he came back to a state where he could function and return to work, but it was clear that this recovery was only partial.

He would, he told me, worry about the smallest thing. If he needed to go to the shops for groceries, he'd worry that maybe he wouldn't have enough money to pay for them, or that, worse still, he'd get to the till and find he'd left his wallet at home. Or what if he made his purchase successfully but dropped the receipt on the way out of the store, and was apprehended for shoplifting, unable to prove his innocence? Much of this inner dialogue never reached the open air, and those around him would have been surprised to know how consumed he was.

He existed in a permanent state of anxiety, terrified that something awful was about to happen and he would be unable to escape. He would have enthusiasm for new projects like re-fitting the kitchen, but when confronted with all the boxes of flat-pack cabinets and furniture, he would end up in a foetal position on the sofa, unable to believe he could cope. The problem was not that he couldn't do these things, but that the physical and mental reaction of extreme panic whirled him far from the source of the first twinge of anxiety and into a fear that was deep, dark and entirely out of proportion.

As this story came tumbling out of him, I realised that it hadn't even occurred to him that this level of ongoing stress could in any way be connected to his low sperm count.

After the first few sessions where he talked and started to make connections, he told me he that felt filled out from the inside for once, not just hollow. And he also talked about the first time he experienced the intense anxiety. When he was seven, his father had left him and his mother and two sisters, and as a little boy had felt a huge responsibility as the new "man" of the house. He felt his mother expected too much of him, and he took on responsibility for everyone in the home being well and happy. That precocious responsibility was probably the reason his employers at the tech company snatched him up, but it was also just a well-developed cover for the seven-year-old boy who needed comfort and reassurance. When that cover began to crack, he broke down.

After a year of regular treatment and support, and a significant improvement in his general well being, his sperm count had bounded up, and he and his girlfriend conceived their first child.

Sometimes people will, out of habit, create brand new burdens for themselves, seemingly as a distraction from their current problems. It's not an easy process even if some kind of therapy is there to support you. It really is a discipline to stop your mind from drifting back into your "story" and making fear or regret your default setting.

It is an uncomfortable truth that we humans create and can carry around a lot of guilt, fear and other negative emotions. Heartache seems to be part of our natural make up, and even if there's nothing present in our day-to-day life to make us suffer, we will go out and find it. We're good at punishing ourselves and others, and many of us have well-crafted and sophisticated ways to create new burdens; hale and hearty parents who can't look after themselves, partners who will never understand us, a father we don't need but desperately want present. We get used to the dark and say we're "fine" when we're carrying around a

heavy load of emotional baggage, which stops us being
who we really are and living our lives to the full.

Being in the Moment

So often our personal story with its full load of unresolved psychological baggage and an inability to "be in the moment" are intertwined. We define who we are by our story. It's impossible to root yourself in the present when you're drunk with thoughts and emotions from the past or longing for something in the future. By getting rid of old problems and curbing your fantasies you sober up and free yourself to be in the present moment and be your self, as you really are. Acupuncture, at a very basic physical level, can bring this kind of awareness because the needle is a physical object going directly into an acupuncture point and focusses your attention right there - right now. This momentary intervention, which immediately affects and balances the flow of energy, has a spontaneous homeostatic knock on effect throughout the body, mind and spirit. This tangible response to treatment is echoed in many of the case studies portrayed in this book, although each experience is unique to that person, but it shows how everyone can access their true self regardless of their current problems or difficulties.

Taoist philosophy tells us our natural and permanent state is one of contentment and peace, and is indestructible. This state lies at the core of every-thing and is the essence of humanity. Some people call this the "God within", but whatever name you want to give it, the important thing to remember is that it is not something you have to find or create; it exists at the heart of all of us. The challenge for you is to raise this consciousness from under the layers of your stories and illusion created by your thoughts and feelings.

I often try to educate patients on this when I see them worrying and fretting about all kinds of things. They look at me as if I am mad and then give me more reasons why they feel so terrible. They're married to misery. That is not to say there are no real problems in life, just as in the natural world there are disasters but the root of existence is one of stillness, peace and love.

So how do we connect with this blissful state? Turn your back on what you see as your problematic life and pay attention to what truly exists within you. It is an act of faith. We talk about "my life" or "my problems" as if they are our possessions that we carry on our backs and make us feel like somebody and oh-so-very important. We take the events around us far too seriously and worse still find our identity through them. Most of the time we believe in the struggle our mind and ego would have us believe is the only way.

Being in the moment or coming to your senses, means exactly that – fully feeling and experiencing what is going on at the moment. For example, if you stop thinking for a second you will be aware of the chair beneath your legs, the smells in the room, and the colours around you. Being consciously present as we live each moment of our lives is grounding and reassuring, and connects us with the "blissful state". Whereas too much thinking and too much agonising can take us off to imaginary places that destabilise us and distract us from the reality of the moment.

If Only...

"If only we had started trying for a baby five years ago". "If only I had not had that termination, my child would now be fifteen". "If only I had played tennis and not rugby and not got kicked in the - you know where". "If only I had started IVF earlier". "If only I had heard about you earlier". "If only we had enough money for egg donation". "If only he would stop smoking".

In our culture playing the "if only" game, much like engaging in gossip, can feel compelling and attractive, but in truth it is something we do to avoid living in the present moment. "If only" takes us backwards and forwards, visiting the past that has gone and the future that doesn't exist, but actually serves no purpose. It just gives us a faux "experience" which brings more pain and keeps us further from being true to ourselves.

My patient Indra must be the "Princess of Stories" who "once upon a time a long time ago" came to tell her tale. She was 33 when she first arrived at my clinic with the story of her life so well formed in her mind and so convincingly delivered that I was seduced into becoming a character in the story too. She pinned her hopes on me to ensure her tale would have "a happy ever after" ending, and I became the fertility Wizard with a flowing cloak and a pointy hat.

Her well-crafted tale told the sad story of the young Indra held hostage by her evil parents. Locked away from the temptations of the 1970s disco revolution, she wept most nights until one day a handsome young man named Paresh appeared at her door selling "spot the ball" coupons. This fateful night was the beginning of one of the greatest love stories of all time, and after weeks of wooing, she was climbing out of a window to scale her garage roof and join him on his round and setting up all sorts of clandestine meetings. These meetings went on for over a year until one night she waited by her window and Paresh did not come. She waited all night, too terrified to imagine what might have become of him, but he never came again.

This was the story she carried around like a favourite book tucked under her arm. Every time she came to see me she would find some way of taking us back there adding new detail and colour and reliving the tragedy and pain of this tale. The true end of the story, which was regularly omitted by Indra until I insisted she tell me what really had happened, was that she had fallen pregnant and promptly told Paresh, hoping that he would be her Prince Charming and rescue her from her castle. In fact she never heard from him thereafter. She had had a termination and told no one what had happened. Indra finally left home aged 28 and had been alone until she met her current partner two years later. They had been trying for a baby ever since.

Indra put an enormous amount of energy into her story, breathing life into it every time she told it. It was important for her to maintain it and nurture it like a child. The amazing thing about her storytelling skill was that each time I heard it, it had a freshness and vitality as if it had all happened yesterday. She also had a story about the future: the house she and her husband would buy and the children they would have, all told with the same zest. The one story she did not have was the one about her present. She seemed unable to relate anything to the here and now. Uninterested in her relationship and work, having few friends and no hobbies, she would do anything to avoid talking about who, what and where she was right now.

During the course of treatment I encouraged her to start identifying how she was feeling right there in the room. I would ask her what she was doing today and would gently bring her back to the present each time as she attempted to pull me into her stories of the past and future.

As treatment progressed Indra began to look more closely at her life and told me how she had started to make changes in her routine, moving from full-time to a four-day week at work, inviting friends to her house and starting an exercise routine. All of these things, rather than simply achieving a better work/life balance, served to bring her focus back to the present moment and the reality of her current life. It was fascinating to feel the change in her as the grip of her stories started to weaken and after three months she never mentioned them again, being far more excited to recount the fun of her daily life.

Conception happens in a moment. It is an event that mirrors orgasm where everything appears to stop for an imperceptible moment, rendering us unable to think and only feel, as we are reminded of what it is like to be truly present. Indra came into her moment and conceived in the same month that she had her first orgasm, six months after starting treatment. She delivered this rather personal piece of information to me as she slipped back to her story for a moment, and rather embarrassedly and gratefully attributed her pregnancy to "the man in the pointed hat".

Faith

Indra clearly trusted me and followed my suggestions. In a sense she surrendered her will to try something new and it worked. Is that what is meant by faith? The confident belief in the truth? Some kind of religious following? In this context it is the willingness to give up control, but that doesn't mean doing nothing and equally it doesn't mean relinquishing control to anyone else. In my experience, most people who have "failed" to conceive feel that they have no other option than to take control and do something about the situation. This at first brings a temporary sense of relief but very soon as each new strategy fails desperation and fear dominate the picture. This of course further exacerbates the problem. It's like being in a maze with no way out.

Whether we accept it or not, we all have that capacity to have faith. Some believe in the power of their vitamin pills, their own intellect, the skill of their doctor or the magic of the acupuncture needles; some in God. Faith is part of being human and it is not prescriptive but its essence is rooted deep within us.

When things go wrong, like finding out you can't get pregnant; this perceived wrongness compounds our illusion of separateness and we are drawn to feeling alone in the world and having to work it all out for ourselves; "If we can just keep control we will be OK" we think. Our doubts, cynicism and fear of anything greater than us is a natural reaction, but just a construct of our mind, the domain and voice of the self made ego that will tell us anything to survive.

If you ask any human being what ultimately they want, you always end up with the same answer: to be happy. To live spontaneously and let go of the idea that we are somehow in control of achieving happiness takes a great leap of faith. We are conditioned to believe that "happiness" is out there somewhere; to be found in a car or a job or a child. In our bid to maintain this illusion of control, rather than find the happiness that already exists within us and see life unfold we find temporary comfort by constructing our own confident belief in what we see as the truth and then find others that will collude with our story to strengthen our case. This rather clumsy and exhausting strategy to be happy and to achieve the things we believe we need is rife in our culture and now even extends to making babies.

First Person: Juliet

"I'd had my first son when I was 34 and my second at 36, and both times my husband and I conceived almost at the first attempt. It never crossed my mind that I might have problems with my fertility, but I had been interested to read a series of features in a women's magazine about Gerad and the stories of women who'd been to his clinic. Each article seemed to encourage a wave of new people willing to try acupuncture, and then a new article covering the successful treatments.

Acupuncture wasn't something I'd considered anyway, as I didn't think it fitted with my faith as a Christian – I just thought it was a bit hocus-pocus. One of the women interviewed was a Christian and had IVF after trying for a baby for years, and her whole church had prayed for her. It was interesting, but I didn't think it concerned me directly.

About a year later I was in a different position. My husband had wanted to try for a third child, but we hadn't had the same luck. I had had a major health scare and was told by my doctors to avoid pregnancy for a while, but when I was given the all clear my head just felt messed up. I wasn't sure if I really wanted a third child in case it affected my career badly, and I'd have to re-jig my life entirely. There was a lot going round in my head.

I had some therapy, which helped, but one day I decided to go and talk to Gerad, because I felt something was wrong with my fertility system. I was a bit nervous about going, and I remember walking in to the treatment room as a Christian and there were all these Buddhas everywhere and thinking, "God, do you want me to do this?" In the end I said a brief prayer and said, "God, I give this session to you." I actually ended up talking a lot about faith with Gerad. He's a trained psychotherapist so he's very easy to talk to, and the first few sessions felt just like chat therapy. The needles didn't do anything in particular until the fourth visit, when he put one point in and it just felt like a pane of glass fell away.

It was as though I'd been wearing these glasses that told me "you've had a really successful career, why are you trying for a baby?" and it was as though my body took over and said, "I'm mad! Why am I compromising my fertility thinking about my career when I really do want a baby?" I discovered that it really did matter to me that I had another child. The next month I found that I was pregnant.

I found that after the baby, my third son, was born when I was 39, I really did want a fourth child, and this time it was the strongest I'd ever felt about having a baby. I'd always thought children would be part of my life, but it hadn't been till my husband suggested we started trying for our first, that it occurred to me to get on with it. The emotions this time round were very different.

Unfortunately, my husband was going through his own crisis at this time, because of the credit crunch which affected his business badly. I couldn't even begin to put pressure on him, even though I knew he wanted a fourth child. One part of me was really angry because I felt he'd called the shots with all of our children, and now he was in control of the situation again, and here was me approaching 40. I'd gotten preoccupied with the idea that 40 was my last chance, and I was desperately craving another child.

The anger was replaced by guilt when my husband recovered and gave the green light, because I thought I was too old and that I was just greedy to want to have another child when so many others couldn't have one. I had friends who were struggling to conceive, and in my wider family were people going through terrible, anxious times.

I was still seeing Gerad, who kept me on an even keel, but we were still not conceiving. When I reached my 41st birthday I gave up. Someone suggested I took *an AMH test, a new fertility test that could show how many eggs I had left and though I didn't think it could do any good, I did it anyway. The result was a level of 7, which is low but above the threshold where they recommend IVF.*

This time it was a much more gradual process. I felt very much at peace, and I really just surrendered and decided it wasn't up to me to try and control things. When I thought of my fertility, I put it in God's hands and thought that what would be would be. I was shocked – and delighted – to get a positive pregnancy test the next month.

I think the connection between mind and body in conception is absolutely fascinating. I know that acupuncture made a huge difference to me, and I don't think it's "magic". For me it's been quite a spiritual thing. It's not like prayer, where you're talking directly to God, but it does give you a sort of stillness in yourself, and that brings you back in line with your faith. I saw Gerad the week before I conceived my fourth child, and I remember going into the session feeling very angry with God, and being embarrassed because I didn't know why I felt that way. I came out feeling very humble and couldn't believe I'd been so worked up before.

We live in a world of laptops and WIFI and we're so full on, and rather than being swept away by that raging torrent of city life where you're bringing up your children and juggling work, the needles seem to restore that stillness in your soul where you connect to God."

Stop Trying

Everyone has heard the example of the couple trying for a baby for years and years before finally deciding to adopt. Within months of happily settling into new parenthood, a natural pregnancy occurs. I have heard this story recounted so many times by patients who are hoping for a family, and yet when I suggest they think about how this example might help them to look at conception from a different point of view, they usually glaze over or think that I am literally suggesting that they adopt.

Every day in my practice I hear people who have been diagnosed with unexplained infertility telling me how long they have been 'trying' to get pregnant. Trying to do anything takes effort and often the exhausted look on people's faces as they recount the numerous cycles of trying to conceive tells a weary tale. Here is our dilemma.

We used to use the term, 'to fall pregnant' because we recognised that it was an involuntary act. We cannot think our way into conceiving just as we cannot think ourselves into falling in love.

We're told time and time again that if we want something we have to knuckle down and fight for it, to organise and rally our resources and push ourselves to our limits to chase that reward. It is absolutely true of many things achieved in life, but it doesn't mean it is the best way to do it. The things which truly are magic in life are the things we have no control over: falling asleep, falling in love, falling pregnant. Three absolutely basic things that in absence can derail your quest for a perfect life, while seeming ludicrously easy for others.

These three fundamental realities of life happen when we are not trying because they are rooted in the part of us that has no conscious choice. There is a part of humanity that must submit to the will of nature and accept that something deep inside us has the ultimate say. The ancient Chinese recognised that just as they had no control over the movement of the Earth and the perceived rising and the setting of the sun, they equally had no control of their waking and sleeping, and so they surrendered to the natural forces and accepted their place as part of nature. This extended to their understanding of fertility; building on the knowledge of nature, when some years the seeds would grow and flourish producing a strong harvest and other years they would struggle to survive.

In the West we've been conditioned to think we're in control; we'll persuade ourselves into a relationship with a partner who never really "clicked", we'll nod off with sleeping pills, and we'll conceive on target just when we want to. But for all our medical innovations, I see couples who have experienced a baby eluding them time and again, only to conceive just when they had given up hope and relaxed.

Wanting something can be dangerous. By that I don't mean that it's wrong to want a particular thing, or that you should think that you don't deserve something, but that the act of truly yearning and obsessing over it can create a tension which is counterproductive to the very goal you're trying to achieve. How do we actively engage in a process that we're desperate to work, while accepting that the matter of conception is out of our hands?

The idea of stopping is terrifying to people. They have been trying to have a child for so long with such diligence and focus that they think that longed for pregnancy is just around the corner. It's like someone who has always chosen the same lottery numbers, and won't change them in case next week is the one when they come up.

To stop trying suggests the end of the road, and all options exhausted, but it's more like a respite. This break and shift of focus is often the beginning of a shift in energy that allows something in you to finally move and change after years of restriction by your own earnest, commendable but often exhausting efforts.

Falling pregnant is about trusting and believing it could happen; we need to get out of the way so that the potent forces of nature can move through us and do what is needed.

First Person: Charlotte

"We weren't trying to have our oldest son, Thomas. I knew I had endometriosis as it had been diagnosed six months before Tim and I got married. We'd been told that conception might be a problem but at that point I wasn't fussed about having children and it didn't really bother either of us whether we had kids or not.

I struggled to get my head round it when I first found out I was pregnant but my life would have gone down a very different path if I hadn't had Thomas. I was working in the fashion business and for want of a better word I was a cold-hearted workaholic bitch! I was motivated by money, fast cars and nice holidays. Looking back now, I suppose I wasn't a very nice person. Having him triggered the maternal instinct, and it softened me around the edges, making me a very different person. It was like having a carrot dangled in front of you; I thought, "If this is what it's like having a boy, imagine what it would be like to have a girl too!".

When Thomas was a couple of years old we started trying for a second child, without thinking it would be difficult, but we had no luck. My first reaction was anger and frustration. There was very little out there for couples going through secondary infertility and I found that a lot of people were unsympathetic. Even my own mother couldn't see why we were so set on having another child; she thought we should be happy with what we had. I can remember walking around the supermarket and seeing mums screaming at their five children with filthy clothes and running noses and thinking "This is unfair!". I was so angry that I almost felt like running over and physically hurting them.

It was really odd dealing with those extreme feelings because the only time I'd felt emotions like that was from a business perspective in the cut-throat world of work! A friend was going through fertility treatments for a first child at the same time as me, and she was treated very sympathetically, but we were just supposed to deal with it.

The drug I was taking, Clomid, makes you feel like you're living with the worst PMT in the world, permanently. I imagine it made me very difficult to live with – well, I know that's true! Physically it was dreadful, but mentally I felt like I was doing something, so every time I got off the hormonal rollercoaster I just wanted to get right back on it again, but I had a husband, friends and family who could see what it was doing to me.

After several unsuccessful rounds of IUI with Clomid, they switched me to gonadotrophin drugs, and that's when the fun starts, because you start having the injections and I can remember that feeling of my ovaries throbbing 24/7 and horrible bloating where you can't get your clothes done up any more. We had intra-uterine insertion, when the sperm is gathered and then injected directly into your womb at ovulation, and after they'd put the sperm in, there was cramping because my uterus was aggravated. I think we had nine or ten rounds of IUI altogether. On the sixth or seventh I got to day 90 after insemination without having a period but although I had pregnancy symptoms, my tests came back negative.

My GP was concerned because there was a slim chance that I had conceived, but that the embryo was developing ectopically, although when I went for a scan it revealed instead that I had polycystic ovary syndrome, and that was why I hadn't had a period for so long. The consultant I saw suggested ovarian drilling, in which the surgeon makes between five and ten holes in the ovary; a process that is supposed to regulate your cycle, although no one knows how it works.

I remember walking down to the operating theatre not thinking anything of having holes drilled in my ovaries. I didn't question anything because I always felt like I was being proactive and that if I did enough procedures we'd find the right one and I would conceive.

I used to use fertility support group message boards on the Internet and although they were really helpful, they also made me impatient because you could see women who'd had the same treatments at the same time and even at the same clinic as you and were producing more eggs, or better quality eggs that could be frozen. My eggs were never good enough for freezing, and people who were able to freeze their embryos didn't have to go through as many doses of fertility drugs.

I measured everything in life in the cost of a night's worth of fertility drugs, at £200 a time. We had several tipping points financially when my husband, Tim would say, "Charlotte, we really can't borrow any more money." We stopped having holidays, we stopped going out, and we started rationing what we bought at the supermarket. I'd always been used to buying nice clothes having worked in fashion, and suddenly I was getting everything in Tesco. You adapt your whole life around it. You don't realise what it's like until you're halfway through it, and then you can't stop.

The crisis came when I got ovarian hyperstimulation syndrome and had to be rushed into hospital. I was very, very sick, and was more swollen than I'd been when I was seven months pregnant with Thomas. I can still see my mum next to my hospital bed saying, 'Charlotte, you are going to kill yourself and you've got a little boy who needs you. Please, please will you stop all this.'

For me that was a real low mentally and physically, the absolute pits. We were at the end of our tether. We had no money to do anymore. I felt wrecked. I'd put on two stone because of all the drugs I'd been taking for years, and I felt I had no marriage left. I knew I was being a bad mother. Poor Thomas was being dragged around to my scans with me. I'd pick him up after school and he'd come to the clinic with me and sit there counting my follicles!

It's a very weird set up that you find yourself in, and I was almost ready to give up, but I remember begging my husband to let me have one more go. He was reluctant, and I said, "Don't worry, they know about the hyperstimulation now; they'll be really careful and I'll know what to look out for. If I don't do it I'll go mad".

One of my friends spotted an article on Gerad in Eve magazine which was all about a journalist who'd had problems conceiving. Apart from the acupuncture, Gerad had advised her to do what she'd always wanted, which was to buy a cat. Soon after she got the cat, she conceived. We'd been in talks to take part in a documentary by Sir Robert Winston on infertility, and when we had lunch with one of the researchers I mentioned that I was considering acupuncture and she told me she'd heard good things about Gerad. As soon as I got home I phoned to make an appointment. I was very skeptical, and Tim was even more so, but I had an *idea that it might help with more IUI treatments.*

I remember walking into the treatment room at Gerad's clinic, and I don't think I even said hello to him, I just said, 'Don't turn round and tell me I need to get a kitten, because I don't really like animals.' I can still picture his face, thinking, 'Jeez, we've got a right one here.

He often reminds me about that first session, because he says I was all, 'I want a baby, except I don't want a baby, I want a girl, and she's got to have curly hair and a little nose that's all stuck up at the front here and she's wearing a pink babygrow with a lace collar and I'm not giving up until I've got her!' And he was probably sitting there thinking, 'and you won't!'

He explained that we'd try to get me through one natural cycle without drugs and once I'd had a period, and gotten into my next cycle, I could try IVF if I wanted, but that I might not still want to go on with it and to take a bit more time instead. I replied that he was lucky I was even giving him one natural cycle, and how he didn't slap me and tell me to go away, I have no idea!

I demanded to know what I needed to do if I didn't need to get a cat, and he just said, 'You just need another focus in life, Charlotte.' That statement really struck me. Afterwards I walked out of the clinic to the Tube and phoned Tim, and said, 'You know, it's really weird.' And he said, 'What's weird?' 'I don't know, but I feel really weird, and do you know? It doesn't really matter if we don't have another baby because everything's going to be all right.' I think Tim thought

Gerad must have drugged me or something! When we were sitting in the kitchen having dinner that night he said, 'Will you talk me through this process?' He thought I'd been hypnotised and I had to reassure him that we'd just talked and I'd had the needles stuck in.

At this stage I think I thought of Gerad as just a nice chap you could pop along and chat to, so it was more like psychotherapy than anything else. I didn't feel anything in particular when the needles were applied.

In the small hours of the morning after my second session I woke up leaking breast milk. My nighty was soaked with it. It was over ten years since Thomas had been born, and I hadn't breastfed him. It was like when you're breastfeeding and haven't expressed any milk for eight hours, and then the baby cries and sets it off. I went to bed feeling completely normal, and woke up at two am to this. That's when I realised that the acupuncture was having a physical effect. There's no way I can make milk leak from my breasts because of something psychosomatic. It shifted my whole mindset.

A couple of weeks later I was cleaning out the garage and something odd happened. I realised that I was starting my period. Every period I'd had before then had begun with 48 hours of agony because of my endometriosis, so I hadn't guessed that I was about to menstruate. It was my first ever pain-free period, and for me it just compounded what had happened with the milk. It couldn't have stopped being painful randomly just after I'd just happened to spontaneously lactate.

I was ready to start the drugs which would regulate again, but at the next session with Gerad, when he was *checking my pulses, he told me to go home and try a pregnancy test because he thought it had finally happened. I used to buy pregnancy and ovulation tests on the internet in bulk in those days and when you've peed on as many sticks as I had, and never seen the double blue line, it's really strange when you see it. I did three tests in a row, and they all came up positive. I decided they must be wrong because they were cheap, so I rushed out to the supermarket and bought several more, and they all had double blue lines too.*

I didn't really believe it till my scan, and my pregnancy was nerve-wracking because I had bleeding throughout. I kept on seeing Gerad and Max was born at 39 weeks, to our delight. Five months after Max was born, I was at Gerad's clinic complaining that my boobs hurt and I felt odd, and that if I didn't know better I'd say I was pregnant, and he checked my pulses and said, "Well, I think you are!". "I can't be!". Well, I was, and that was my little girl, Clementine, so you can imagine that by the time she was born I thought I'd won the lottery.

Five-Element acupuncture has changed my life and not just because I was able to have children after that long journey. It's made me a much better person. It's made me really look at how I am. Six years ago I was angry about life, full stop. I did fight it because I thought I didn't want to change too much of who I was, and he said, 'Look, you're always going to be feisty, we're never going to take that away from you, but just learn to channel it.' I'd blocked everyone and everything out of my life and become this hugely focussed – well, almost a machine – person who ram-raided her way through life. I definitely have more of a cup half full rather than cup half empty attitude now. I've changed jobs to work with an organisation which arranges international exchanges for students, which uses my old business skills but also gives me a chance to help look after teenagers who are far from home and sometimes quite troubled. It feels worthwhile in a way that my old management career never did. It can be tough with three children, especially when two are just thirteen months apart, but I count my blessings every day."

For someone like Charlotte or Juliet to let go of control can be an incredibly liberating and powerful experience and can have surprising results. To accept that the struggle no longer helps you and that you are best served by surrendering to or giving up whatever it is you are fighting for, is an act of faith in trusting that by taking the path of least resistance something will change for the better. It is not about losing – far from it - it's just about having the humility to accept your place in the world. Along the way you might discover life-changing things about yourself, as Charlotte did. Charlotte was totally distracted by her new baby when she accidently conceived her longed for little girl. She certainly was not "trying" at that point.

This is where things get tricky. Anything we try to achieve where the decision is made from our head is less likely to work out well. Good decisions are not a calculated thought but the outcome of a complex internal process unknowable by our conscious mind.

Often we wake in the morning and somehow we know to change something or without even realising we find ourselves doing something differently. As I mentioned earlier our minds are wonderful instruments when used correctly but pale into insignificance in the presence of our "true self" when it comes to knowing what is best for us. Being yourself and living in a way that is congruent with who you are and what you love taps into something greater than you could ever imagine. "But I would love a baby", I hear you cry. "Is that not true for me and who I am?" Yes, of course, but now consider leaving that thought alone, enjoy your life as it is today and change what you know you can and leave the rest alone.

A couple who came to see me called Andrew and Catherine lived a very safe life. They had jumped through all the right hoops, graduated from the right universities, secured good jobs and bought a flat with a reasonable mortgage so that they could save some money every month. When I first saw them for treatment, I was struck by the sensation of claustrophobia that rose off them both. It wasn't just that they seemed trapped, they were also resentful and they kept chiming, "disappointed". They had been told to be sensible and that this would bring its' own reward.

As a practitioner it's my job to stay neutral and not pass judgment on the lives of patients. After all, if I've learned anything over the years of working with people, it's that every individual and couple is unique and needs to find their own way of living. Andrew and

Catherine's life would have been perfect for plenty of other people but it clearly wasn't right for them. I asked Andrew, "If this is the route of your choice, what does the outcome tell you?" and he simply said, "It ain't working."

After that we talked about what they could do to change things. I continued treating Andrew and one of my colleagues started seeing Catherine. We didn't make any specific suggestions but continued with treatment and hoped this would relieve that sense of claustrophobia. After a while, they made a decisive swerve off the track.

They sold their modest little house and took out a whopping mortgage on a new place on the outskirts of London with a lot of work to do. They told me with glee that they'd lied to their parents about the extent of the debt they'd taken on, and threw themselves into doing up the house. They'd been dying to get out of town for a while but had put the move on hold till they had a child. Now, despite the stress of an imprudent mortgage, they began to enjoy themselves. At weekends they were out at flea markets and antique dealers, picking up all kinds of oddities for the house. There was something uncharacteristically extravagant and theatrical about this new joint project. They even asked where my paint supplies for the clinic came from, because they fancied a gold ceiling. They raided their sacrosanct savings fund and took an extravagant holiday because they had no idea why they'd been saving up in the first place. Their lives seemed to flesh out and fill with colour, literally. Where before they'd told me that they'd only ever gone out on Friday and Saturday nights, they now started going out on a Monday or a Wednesday, and staying out late instead of rushing back to bed for an early night. Instead of waking up shattered and hung-over, they were surprised to find they had more energy.

With all this new life, they had stopped focussing on having a child, and when Catherine had a positive pregnancy test it seemed incidental to the rest of their news about the house and the new furniture they'd found that weekend. It had become the most normal, natural thing in the world.

A Fresh Perspective

Choosing a job, a lifestyle or when to start a family or in fact anything in life, is exactly that; a choice. This for the most part feels conscious and deliberate – but is it? There are also thousands of tiny unconscious choices, made every day of our lives that either resonate with or move further from our own true nature, and every time we choose something in life we are playing out our own story or as the Chinese saw it – fulfilling our destiny. We can see this as a tremendous freedom at its best, but how do we know or make sure those choices and decisions are being made from the right part of our selves?

We put a lot of energy into clinging to choices we have made in our heads, being attached to what we have created and believe to be right. Very often we have invested years of hard work and determination to achieve our goals and we will not give them up lightly even when we know our experience of them is hollow and empty. If we get stuck we will stagnate, or fail to realise how discontented we've become. Problems with jobs, workmates or family seem insurmountable, but they only are if we let them.

We need to be flexible in life and open to inevitable change. Even the most organised, according-to-plan existence can be derailed by a great misfortune or a lucky chance. I believe it's as possible to conceive a baby at forty as at twenty if we're prepared to change and adapt with the passing of time and maintain our physical, mental and spiritual well-being throughout life.

One couple who came to see me, Ann and Scott, thought ahead to plan the lifestyle they wanted. They had started a buy-to-let business because they thought it would give them freedom to enjoy their lives without being chained to a desk or employed by someone. They had been very successful and were now ready to have children, but something was wrong.

Ann wanted to have children as she was in her late thirties and running out of time, she thought. Scott was less rushed. When pushed, in a single session without Ann, he admitted that he wanted to maintain the freedom they'd hoped for when they set up their business. He said he wouldn't try though, because Ann wanted them to get on with having a baby now.

After a little more thought and some shaking up, the two of them decided to take a year off from the baby conveyor belt and hired someone to look after their business for twelve months. They took off for Canada, got hold of a Winnebago and traveled all the way to Chile. Ann hadn't been as keen as Scott but she took the risk and ended up loving the trip. They conceived their first child in Brazil at Mardi Gras.

People often tell me they can't leave a job which makes them miserable. That statement just digs their pit a little deeper. I'm not anti-career, and I definitely don't think that women need be out of the office and back in the kitchen to conceive, but I am suggesting there is a balance to be struck between work and life, and for everyone to develop their ability to sound out who they are and what works for them.

I remember watching a friend of mine who was

hoping to get pregnant go through a real renaissance after realising that her life in London was intolerable and maybe affecting her fertility. She was 40 at the time, living in a dingy basement flat with a younger boyfriend whom she adored, and teaching an oversize class of demanding children, many of whom came from deprived backgrounds. Worn out and tired, she'd half convinced herself that her boyfriend was bound to leave her for someone else, and no amount of reassurance helped her see how ridiculous that was.

She'd slipped into bulimia, and as friends we were all worried about her because she was getting thinner and thinner.

In the end she didn't sign herself up for therapy, counselling or acupuncture. She took up her boyfriend's suggestion that they move to his home country of Spain and begin a new life. They moved to a tiny village where he got a job in the local tourist industry and she freelanced as an English teacher for local kids. They had time to hike into the mountains every day and Ann, who is a country girl at heart, blossomed. When I visited them I could hardly recognise her as she looked like a different woman. They had no problem conceiving their first child, only three months after relocating.

There's no absolute right or wrong; you have to take action and do things in your own way. That might mean at times being completely inert or manic, it doesn't matter, as long as you are firmly rooted in the part of you that is content and at peace. In the constant flux of life, when you follow your true path your "pendulum" is able to return to the balancing point, the middle, and not stay at one swing of the polarity or the other, and that's what will keep you safe, well and in the fertile zone. When people start to live this way you see all kinds of health benefits. They sleep a little better, enjoy exercising, feel more at peace, have more fun, and whilst enjoying being who they are, finally conceive.

If something is not working then change surely is a solution. The hardest part is working out what needs to change and how to do it. It takes a great deal of courage to take an honest look at ourselves and be prepared to change the things we think are right but know deep down are wrong and are making us sick and unhappy. Real choice does not come from the mind but from the spirit. A choice is something we feel in ourselves, our bodies; our instinctive compass guiding us as our life unfolds. It is only when we start listening to our self and our truth that we can take full responsibility for the choices we make and the life we lead.

Intention

At the beginning of the first meeting with every patient I ask a simple question; "If you could have anything from this treatment, what would you put at the top of your list?" Very quickly and without a second thought the majority of people inevitably jump and say – "to have a child". My next question is, "why?" I'm really not surprised that most people don't seem to have any specific reason, as our instinct to be loved and have children is wonderful and innately human and not something we need to spend time and effort thinking about.

If I then suggest we imagine the baby is a done deal and ask "But what would you love for yourself?", people are also often lost for an answer as their focus has been almost entirely on becoming a parent for so many years. With a little further prompting and encouragement to step outside of the baby "box" the deeper needs and desires arise and are often quite surprising. There is often a great sense of relief and excitement to think about something else other than conception and the longed for baby, and to further realise that this new focus on self could possibly contribute to helping their "main complaint".

How often do we stop to ask ourselves what we would truly love in our lives, and do we question the things we think we want and intend to get? We just get on with life, and our innate talents and desires either get very confused and mixed in with a whole list of stuff we think we need, or they are forgotten altogether. Of the patients I typically see for fertility, it is easy to make the assumption that their primary intention is to have a child almost to the exclusion of everything else in their life. But if I talk to a couple separately and ask them how they will feel if they are unsuccessful in becoming parents, they will frequently give different responses; one truly devastated, the other taking it in their stride and sure that they will find something else and be fine to go on with life. But is this always the truth?

As we get older and leave the spontaneity of our youth, our "heart's desire" and what we think we "want" both individually and as a couple can become incongruous, resulting in many mixed messages that become apparent as you negotiate the difficult path of fertility treatment and try to manage your relationship along the way.

I often see this with men. They say they want a child, but seem indifferent, and appear to be shrugging their shoulders as if just along for the ride. I don't think there's much room in our culture for men to be over enthusiastic about becoming a parent. For women it's an issue that, like it or not, is brought up throughout their lives, from gifts of dolls to pointed remarks about biological clocks and the constant monthly reminder that your system is preparing for a child. Men, often ignored in fertility clinics and even registered in their partner's name when giving a semen sample, get more involved as they go along. They have the time to think about the process and invest in the idea of having a child. Often when the first round of IVF fails, for example, men surprise themselves as they realise how disappointed they feel.

So what is the significance of this magic word "intention" and how does it help when hoping to conceive? As I said earlier that it was important to "stop trying" to have a baby and just let the process happen, then isn't it contradictory to suddenly talk about "intention"?

Teenagers, you might say, get pregnant without intention all the time, but that's not entirely true. For them "intention" is a clear, primitive drive to get out there and seduce and be seduced and make babies. They don't accidentally fall into bed together. It's very spontaneous, very pure and very powerful, and it works also in older couples in the honeymoon period. "Instinct" is perhaps another term for it; the intention that's the driving force in nature to make things happen. It could be argued that "intention" fuels our libido and powers the drive to conceive.

In the Five-Element system the "mind" or our "intelligence" is the sum total of all the activities of the organs and functions previously described in the section where we looked at each of the five elements. When we are in balance our heart and mind are "one", and our "heart's desire" to have a child is programmed and ever present in all of us. This primal code is set to provide the potential for the survival of our species, however the only way this message can be realised is through "intention".

If you are ready to become a parent in your "head" and on a deeper level your heart is not on board and therefore not in sync, this lack of congruence will jar and could negatively affect the desired outcome. In Chinese philosophy the heart and the uterus are seen as having a very close relationship; the "heart – uterus axis" refers to the heart stimulating ovulation while providing a home and dwelling place for the spirit. Similarly, the uterus becomes the home for the developing child. The ancient Chinese knew that the mind and body alone were not capable of making a baby.

It's taken for granted that generally people want to have children; but your intention, particularly as you get older, will influence and determine the choices you make as you move on from trying naturally, to assisted conception and on again, perhaps, to adoption. Are you open to accepting that your intention has changed? There may come a point in the process when your heart is no longer in it, and you want to turn your focus and the focus of your relationship elsewhere. Does it have to be a child that is biologically both yours and your partners, or even biologically yours at all?

It's not just about having a strategy, but really engaging with your deeper feelings on the matter. Sometimes the block to conception begins in a misplaced, misjudged "intention" that you don't really experience consciously at all.

One couple I see, Steve and Cathy are a good illustration. Steve already has four kids from a previous marriage who are going through their teens and acting out with a vengeance. He's a very full-on character, with plenty of energy and personality and he's always at the centre of his social circle. He's hugely happy with Cathy, who's also extremely sociable and cherished by her friends. Neither is fundamentally troubled in themselves or in their relationship; for all Steve's fireworks, they seem to be very content, except for the fact that they have now begun the conveyor belt of fertility treatment.

Steve thinks Cathy wants a child, Cathy says she does too, but I'm not sure that they are prepared to go through what's required. The main physical problem is that both are extremely overweight and don't do any exercise. This is not in itself a guarantee of infertility, but certainly a factor to be considered if there is a problem with conceiving naturally. My first suggestion would be that they changed their lifestyles and diets and made a few sacrifices of pleasure for the greater pleasure of a baby, but they seem to just want to sweep that under the carpet. They want to have acupuncture and then IVF and maybe ICSI, or an egg donor if that doesn't work.

Their ambivalence about having a child – highlighted to me by the way they overlook the most glaring obstacle – is lost to them because they are dazzled by the list of options available to them at various clinics. They've made a problem where none existed, and fussed over building an elaborate construction of further dilemmas and heartaches out of it. They could go on happily with their lives without changing their weight or their lifestyle, surrounded by friends and family. They could also commit themselves to becoming healthier, and I'm sure they'd conceive then, but at the moment they don't have to take responsibility for their bodies as IVF offers them a distraction and a way to evade their own ambivalence about having a child and health problems. For me as a practitioner success wouldn't necessarily be Cathy getting pregnant, but both of them improving their health and getting body in as fine fettle as mind and spirit.

In contrast to Cathy and Steve's ambivalence, my patient Eve, whose focussed intention and willingness to do whatever it takes was clearly apparent in her journey to have another child.

Eve – *"I have a daughter who is now twenty one, and when she was four I had a second child, a little boy, who sadly died four days after he was born, and we were devastated. He'd had the equivalent of a massive stroke in utero a few days before he was born, but nobody knew why, and we were told to wait eighteen months before trying again.*

We were very fortunate to get pregnant again and I had very good care, and my second son was born without problems. Everything was fine, but I still felt as though there was a gap. I didn't need to replace my first son; I just felt very strongly that there was a space for someone else. I didn't act on it, but got on with my career and kept myself busy, but when I was forty the feeling came back more strongly than ever.

We talked long and hard about having a fourth child, but when we tried, nothing happened. After a few years I started having acupuncture and within three months I was pregnant, but I had loads of stress at the time – my father and my best friend were dying, and I was racing between them – and I miscarried for whatever reason at two months.

By this time I was 44 or 45 and very aware that I was really pushing it, and running out of time. We decided that the best thing was to give up and to adopt a British child, and began the interviews and home tests required. The agency were delighted to have us as mature parents and said that everything should go well when we turned in a huge stack of references. The children and we were interviewed repeatedly and it all went swimmingly until we were within months of being given a child.

The agency called me at work and said there was a problem. In one of the interviews my son had said that he didn't mind what a new child in the family looked like, as long as they didn't act like the very disturbed son of a friend of ours, who was very hyperactive. That raised a flag. Just like that, the agency rescinded everything, and we were back where we'd started.

Acupuncture helped keep me sane during all this heartbreak, but I didn't think we had any chance of filling that gap in the family. That was when Gerad suggested using an egg donor. I was still fit and healthy and didn't think I would have a problem carrying a child. I just thought that my eggs were too old, and it would be irresponsible to use them.

Once we'd found a good clinic, everything flew by. In only a few months we were sent details of all the potential donors, which was really quite odd. The clinic was in America and all the women had such glamorous headshots, and it was bizarre, like supermarket *shopping. There were lists of their college degrees and so on. You never get a chance to talk to them, and you think you should take a long time choosing, but at the same time you have the clinic telling you that you have to make up your mind by Wednesday!*

Eventually we chose a donor and my husband flew to the States to give his sample; he flew in one day, did the business and flew out the next. He said it was the most bizarre thing he'd done in his whole life! Gerad had been treating me to make sure I was in peak condition, and I flew over to have the embryo implanted a few days later, before returning home. I had a very smooth pregnancy and the NHS was brilliant about it. There was no judgement at all, and they were all incredibly supportive. Our son was born nine months later, when I was 50 – this precious, chatty little boy who brings so much joy to all of us.

I never felt weird about adopting or using an egg donor. I love babies, and I love children, and I just didn't feel it would be an issue. I think you have to be a pretty tough person to go through it though, because you're putting yourself through a lot. I already had two healthy children so I could be a teeny bit pragmatic about it, although of course you put all your hopes in. If it's your last option and you have no child, then it must be agony. I would like more people to think they could do this and think it's not only for really wealthy people. I'm lucky I've been able to explore and fulfill that drive I had."

Intention is all about "showing up" for something that is real; being fully present to whatever it is you hope to achieve without the need or desire to "make" it to happen. Ambivalence is the opposite. This is a very subtle approach and does get confused with the passive hands-off approach of "Let's just step back and see if it happens", and the determined sheer grit approach of "I will succeed". There's no guarantee for example of finding a partner just because you think you want one; you do at least have to feel something as you get out in the world and meet people. This is also true of fertility – there are no guarantees of success, but there is a lot you can do, as already suggested in this book. A clear and congruent relationship between your heart and mind can make an enormous difference to your hopes and dreams of success.

Gratitude

What I often see as one of the great obstacles to a peaceful and graceful path to having a child is our western mindset and culture of "entitlement". We somehow came up with the idea that we are entitled to so many aspects of our life - including a loving partner and children - and when we don't get them as expected we feel abandoned and lost like small children who cry "It's not fair!". This may sound harsh but most of us have been brainwashed by our collectively created consumer culture, that would have us believe that having and owning more and more is a human right, and only further feeds our sense of entitlement.

When hoping to conceive, my advice to you is to relax, sit back and remember that we are not "entitled" to anything. Life and all it brings is a wonderful gift and every day that we wake up and realise we still even exist is a blissful bonus and not an entitlement. In our culture of "I want" and "I need", we have lost a genuine sense of gratitude for some of the most basic things in life; health being one.

We take our body and mind for granted when things are working well, and we rarely stop to marvel at this complex organism that is our physical form performing most tasks quietly and efficiently and leaving us alone to get on with life. However, as soon as something goes wrong it becomes overwhelming to us, gratitude flies out the window and all those years of great health are forgotten. Fertility - like relationships - is something we feel that we are entitled to, and providing it all works out we simply take it for granted. We become spiritually lazy and with laziness comes unhappiness sucking us straight down the victim shoot where we settle in and begin to believe this is our natural state.

Not only do we expect a perfect mate but we also want the character we have been sold since childhood, and then when it comes to relationship plus baby, it seems that we get even more particular and generally favour the "Mills and Boon" version as being the best way to have a child. Even some of the most liberal and alternative people I know tone down and suddenly morph into Mr and Mrs 1950's Suburbia when the baby making alarm bell rings.

By moving out of "entitlement" and into a place of gratitude for what we have right now (you are still breathing I hope), we immediately soften and synch with the rhythms of nature that are always waiting in the wings for us to step out of the way and provide the very best for all of us; nature's gift of abundance.

The Business

Since the first IVF baby was born in 1978 our attitude to conception has changed. Conception used to be a gift – sought or unsought – from nature, and we had to accept what she chose to deal us. Now you can buy a pregnancy, or at least a chance of one, with medical procedures that give us the illusion of control at every stage. In 2010, two vets in Australia even proclaimed that soon no human would need to have sex to procreate; IVF would take care of all that. Cows had a 100% greater chance of conceiving with artificial methods than natural, they pointed out, and surely the same success was just a hop, skip and a jump in science away from the grasp of humans.

The problem, they admitted, was that for humans, IVF only works in 28.6 per cent of cycles of treatment for women under the age of 35, and as they get older, this measly success rate drops even lower. The Human Fertilisation and Embryology Association's tally for the overall success rate of all medical fertility clinics is just 22 per cent; less than a quarter. Why doesn't it work as well for humans as it does for cattle? Could it be that we're far more complicated beings than cows? Of course. A cow doesn't worry about its relationship, or ending up on its own in old age, or even if there will be food tomorrow or if it wants to change its job and follow its dreams.

Not surprisingly, these vets overlook what makes us human – as do many of the doctors and gurus in the fertility industry – assuming that a human is so simple that you just have to provide the right fodder and work out the correct schedule, and conception will ensue. Failing that, you can add large amounts of hormones to super-enhance the production of eggs, and then give the sperm a special boost by injecting it directly into target. No obstacles, no struggle, no natural selection and, of course, no orgasms.

Some consultants seem to think that if modern medicine can't help them, it's a couples' own fault, and not that of the fertility business. They will drop bombshells on their patients, telling them they have a low chance, or not a chance in hell, and a lot of these people are plunged into despair, for which there's little or no counselling. I'm not opposed to all the incredible advances that have been made in medical technology, and I am happy to help people who have entered into the process. Many people do have physical mechanical problems, such as blocked fallopian tubes or extensive endometriosis that cannot be overcome by clearing up their lifestyle or sorting out their hearts, but I still feel that there's a hole at the core of the business. The state of a patient's spirit is too invisible, and if visible, too time-consuming and complicated and nuanced for a fertility clinic to tackle.

Sometimes, for the prospective parents, it comes down to a catch 22: leave work on time and take an hour or two to relax and recover and balance work and life on the chance that it will help you conceive, or else work those longer hours so you can afford the conveyer belt of treatment and a trip overseas to find an egg donor, all the time with this drumbeat telling you "too late, hurry, hurry!"

Added to the purely physical interpretation of fertility problems is a culture of blame and sniping that thrives in scare stories and the cult of the "biological clock." These "warnings" to women to conceive before it's "too late" are usually accompanied by some science-y statistics that don't hold up so well on examination. One headline screams that most women have lost seven eighths of their 2,000,000 eggs by the age of thirty. If you do the maths, you realise that this average woman still has 500,000 eggs to spare at 30 – even Octomom doesn't need to have 500,000 babies. You only need one egg to have a child, not an omelette's worth.

Some women are told they have too many "natural killer cells" in their uterus, which might be attacking implanted foetuses. Enterprising doctors then suggest a dose of drugs that will knock out their immune system for a while, so the killer cells can't gobble up the new embryo. There is no conclusive proof that uterine natural killer cells do attack embryos, or even that the blood test performed for this "diagnosis" has any bearing on the number of marauding cells in the womb, but of course it sounds dramatic, and I'm sure it terrifies women who are told they are harbouring baby killing organisms!

Lately clinics began to trumpet a new test, for anti-Müllerian hormone levels (AMH), which they said would "predict a woman's menopause" by telling her how many eggs she had left. The result of this, for me, was a flurry of devastated women in my clinic who'd been told they had far too few ova left to conceive.

One woman who, at forty-one, hadn't conceived after two years (a pretty normal span of time, all things considered) went to a one-stop shop fertility clinic, which told her that they would just run some tests. She had no idea what most of them were, and when her results came in, the consultant "gleefully" announced that her AMH level was so low that there was no way she would conceive naturally, so they'd put her straight on the clinic's egg sharing programme. When she expressed her horror and shock, the doctor snapped back, "Well, what do expect when you're over forty?".

She was furious and left immediately, later booking an appointment to begin a course of acupuncture. After six months she had conceived naturally, without any help from the consultant. She believes now that it was a direct result of the acupuncture treatment at our clinic, but I think it may only have played a small role because, aside from her understandable anger with the consultant, she had a healthy, balanced life and outlook. If it took you, say, six months to conceive in your early twenties, that's six rolls of the dice, three years to conceive at 41 is 36 rolls – it may only have been a matter of holding her nerve until the right number came up and the right egg met the right sperm.

Faith had her first child at 36 with no difficulty, but when she got pregnant with her second child three years later, she miscarried at eleven weeks, which was unforeseen and startling for her. She lost some of her confidence in her ability to have a child, and when her husband lost his job and slid into depression, she became increasingly anxious that she would never have another child.

As she'd been told that her greatest chance of conceiving was in the first few months immediately after miscarriage, and as her husband was not mentally in the right place to enthusiastically start making babies, she decided to have an AMH test in order to understand "how long she had left".

The verdict was 0.3% chance. Faith was gutted. She went from a capable, outwardly successful woman to a wreck, and by the time she came to the clinic she had lost half her hair and was running hysterically back and forth between nutritionists, reflexologists and me. I can only say that the only time I've seen such a dramatic depression resulting from a medical diagnosis is in the newly diagnosed HIV positive patients of the early 1990's that I treated at Kings College Hospital. It felt like a death sentence to her. She still had her husband, her home and her daughter, and there was no other proof other than the AMH test to say that she couldn't have another child, but it was as though she could barely hear what was being said to her.

Plenty of people argue that acupuncture only has a placebo effect, but I have never seen a contraceptive placebo as powerful as a low AMH result, delivered without sympathy. Faith went from a woman who had conceived easily twice in her late thirties – supposedly with this 0.3% chance – to "barren". Hopefully it will be possible for her to regain the equilibrium and health she had before she took the test.

The AMH test doesn't tell you what quality of eggs remain, only their quantity. It's also inconsistent – if a woman has more than one AMH test she may get a completely different result each time. Plenty of women who'd been told their eggs were inadequate had absolutely no problems conceiving and others who'd had a positive tick on their clipboard found themselves having difficulty. Meanwhile, another myth about science had sunk into the culture, and the idea that women were racing against the clock was reinforced once more.

Part of the problem is the widespread belief that at birth, a baby girl contains a full set of eggs, ready to start rolling down the fallopian tubes at puberty, and that, if they're not used early enough, then just like chicken eggs in a fridge they will "go off". This is nonsense. You are born with the potential for a certain number of eggs. The quality of those eggs depends on the quality of your over-all health at the time that the egg receives the hormonal signal to mature, prior to erupting from the ovary and heading down the fallopian tubes to your womb.

Even something as apparently simple as sperm testing can be less than straightforward. A sample is taken, the sperm examined under the microscope. How many are there? Are they swimming well? Are they damaged? An assessment is made and the verdict delivered. The man is either given the thumbs up, or emasculated by being told he's the one at fault.

The problem is that it takes sperm three months to mature from first development to ejaculation. In the testicles the naive sperm cells are constantly creating new gametes. Ideally, these will go on growing and developing their tails and nice healthy heads until a batch of 40,000,000 is ready to go a quarter of a year later. In reality, the entire process, even before the sperm are anywhere near a vagina, is natural selection. The cells are very sensitive to their environment, so if, say, you celebrated the new year to the full on December 31st, the sperm that began their lives that day might have been dealt a severe early blow, and struggle. In any case, only 10 per cent of the 40,000,000 have a head that's sufficient to break the walls of the ovum, and only 10 per cent of those have a tail. There's 400,000 left and some of those don't have any genetic material in the head. And then they face that hostile environment, with an inimical pH and all those phagocyte cells. Oh and if the man took his test at the end of March, those soused New Year sperm will give an unfairly poor rating. Perhaps he did a two week detox at the beginning of January. If the clinic tested his sperm again in early April, they might find the microscope slide full of sturdy specimens, and give the same man a clean bill of fertility health.

Worse still, a man with a spectacularly unhealthy lifestyle might happen to have his test three months after a rare dose of sobriety and restraint, with the end result that he unfairly gets the all-clear and his female partner has to go through years of hormonal injections and examinations to work out what's wrong with her. In Western medical history, more emphasis is placed on "curing" and "treating" the female body than the male, often in a way that makes you think "blaming" would be a more appropriate word than treating.

First person: Martin

"One of the first things that was suggested when I went for acupuncture treatment was that I should be tested for a change, and to have 3 tests over a period of 2 months. When we got all the results back it turned out that the problem had been with me all along. I wish that could have been identified earlier because we would have saved ourselves a lot of heartache and waiting. All of that takes an emotional toll and it takes a toll on your relationship too. If I could give any advice to men in the same situation I found myself in, it would be to try to escape that medical focus being just on the woman. I'm sure men feel the same as women who have been told they are infertile – that it's some sort of failure of their sexuality if they can't produce a child – and in some ways the medical profession lets them off the hook by concentrating on women. The men don't have to confront what's going on, and can avoid awkward soul searching. It's not like men are going to be rushing into Internet forums to talk about their low sperm counts! It may feel like there's a lot stacked against taking a holistic perspective, but you have to consider that something is up with you, and take steps to do something, because a lot of implications can follow from the way you're treated. We might have had more children if we'd had that clarity earlier on."

Instead, women are bombarded with this message that it's all their fault. They're selfish if they have babies as teenagers, and selfish if they wait till their forties, selfish if they only have one child, selfish if they have more than three, selfish if they have a high-flying career, selfish if they don't earn enough to support the children. They're using up NHS resources if they have IVF, and state resources if they have a large family. They're told to settle for "Mr Good Enough" instead of holding out for a consuming passion. Ageism and misogyny are packaged in emotive terms like "Russian roulette" and "tragic infertility".

Once you have children, as Lizzie put it, "Everything you do is wrong. I stayed at home with my son because I could work from there and he was so precious to me, but as soon as people find out I only have one child they disapprove. When I was growing up if your mother went out to work it was the same thing. If you have children too young, too late, too quickly, not quickly enough – people pass comment. It's all rubbish and you have to steer your own course. Every family is different."

A childless life is often cast as a sad, wasted one. For those like me who have no kids, that comes as a bit of a surprise, and it's also pretty insulting to be told that your life counts for nothing compared to those who have managed to produce a child. Your relationships, your loves, your home, your career, your contribution to the world, the sum of you as an individual is truly nothing if you haven't had a child? It's a doubtful kind of world to want to live in.

As we've seen in this book, by the time a lot of people reach their later thirties, they no longer understand what "normal" and "healthy" might be for them as they're entrenched in habits or a lifestyle that their body can no longer sustain while simultaneously nourishing a pregnancy. Once that imbalance is corrected, be it physical, mental or spiritual, many "older" women and men go on to conceive. From what I've seen, as long as a woman is menstruating and a man producing sperm, they have a chance to conceive. Why else would nature expend the resources on a menstrual cycle and sperm production? If it can happen naturally, then why judge? If there is a "time bomb" it's the risk we take with our spiritual and physical health overall – not just our genitals and reproductive organs – by not being able to stand back and set ourselves straight.

Success

One of the greatest difficulties in treating patients for infertility is that there is only one perceived successful outcome – a baby. No matter how much I communicate the other benefits of treatment, patients tend to come for one specific reason and this is where their focus remains. This is of course completely understandable but if the job of the acupuncturist is to support and care for all patients equally then there will always be the patients who are not successful in having a child and should not be seen as having failed. The stakes are high for all patients struggling with infertility. It is a very public experience and people not only feel compelled to succeed for their own needs and desires but also the needs and desires of family and friends who have their own set of expectations.

Success can be a very subjective experience. We very quickly set our own challenges in life and set off on a journey where life is about succeeding or failing at those. When I was very young I opened a small business that ran for just over two years. It was moderately successful but felt overwhelming and afforded me little time to socialise. As my interest waned the business started to fail and eventually closed down. At the time I was aware that it was a natural end as it did not serve me and therefore it was appropriate to let it close. However in the eyes of my peers, it was a failure.

I moved to the States shortly thereafter, much chastened. Standing in a supermarket checkout queue one day I started chatting with a man about where I was from and why I had moved. I told him my shameful story, to which he replied, "That's great! Once you've gone bust two more times, then you'll know what you're doing!" This different perspective shifted my thinking and suddenly the demise of my business became a success because it was part of my education.

First person: Dorothy

"I've been trying for almost two years to have a second child. I have polycystic ovary syndrome, and my GP told me it would take three years to conceive a child so we started trying as soon as we were married. Within three months I fell pregnant at 34 and we were totally gobsmacked and delighted. I had a very healthy pregnancy, but our daughter's birth was very difficult, and I caught a very rare Strep C septicaemia infection – I think I was the only woman in the country to have it – and nearly died.

My organs were on the verge of failure and layers of skin came off my hands and feet like a snake. I had to have blood transfusions and the doctors threatened a hysterectomy, although I didn't have to have one in the end. When I got out of the hospital six and a half weeks later, the doctors told me to leave at least a year before trying to conceive a second child, to give my body a chance to recover.

When we first started trying again, I was very stressed for the first six months. Part of it was that I desperately wanted to have a normal birth, and I never wanted my daughter to think that it was because I nearly died having her that she didn't have a brother or

218

sister. A lot of people said they couldn't believe I was even considering going through it all again, but for me it felt as though I would mend something by having a second child.

After nine months, nothing seemed to be happening and I panicked that the infection had done some permanent damage. I went to my GP but she brushed me off and said, "You'll be absolutely fine." Luckily, as I had private insurance I was able to begin a series of tests, but I also started seeing Gerad for acupuncture at the same time, to see if that would help.

For the first four months I was still stressed out. The medical results were coming in and revealing that there was nothing wrong with my husband or I, and to be honest that just made it all the more frustrating. Every time I got my period I'd have a bad few days when the hormones were in full flow and I just didn't get it – what was wrong? Why weren't we getting pregnant? And then you just think, onwards and upwards into the next month!

Acupuncture helped with that. I also started to see a therapist at the same time, and gradually I've got a much more balanced perspective. Now I just want to follow this journey with a more laissez-faire attitude and just let things happen. After each session there is definitely a change in me. I feel very upbeat when I come out of the clinic, after I'd gone in irritable and uptight. He doesn't tell you which point he's using or why, but it feels like a total release.

We haven't conceived naturally as a result of the treatment, but I do feel like I'm a better person for it, *and my husband would definitely say I'm less stressed. I would never have done all this work on myself if we'd been able to have a second child without a hitch, and I think I'm going to be a better mother to my daughter because I'm stronger now and I'm dealing with my issues.*

I do still want a sibling for my girl because I had three sisters and we're all incredibly close, and it's hard to think of her missing out on having that kind of support and friendship. We're embarking on IVF now, and on our first trip to the clinic I felt so much less alone. Suddenly we were surrounded by people who were going through the same thing.

I don't regret not trying IVF sooner, because I'm in a much better frame of mind than I was a year ago before I started seeing the therapist and having acupuncture. I think it would have been horrendous, and hell on the whole family as well, and I wouldn't have been prepared for the fact that it might just not work. It's a formidable prospect because I don't know how the drugs will affect me or if we shouldn't try one more time to have a child naturally, but I feel proud that we lasted two years and didn't just leap in after a few months. It just feels like the right point on our journey, and we'll deal with it as it comes."

In the West we have a relatively fixed idea of good or bad, success or fail, which feels unyielding and restrictive at times. When I first started treating patients for infertility I was also sucked into this success/fail paradigm, which was exciting when treatment resulted in a pregnancy and dispiriting when it didn't. I quickly realised that this pressure and my own emotional investment in success did not serve my patients. My expectations only created more pressure for them.

Life is gentler than this, and, providing we have a good level of mental and spiritual flexibility, what we see as success or failure can just simply be our current state, which is neither "good" nor "bad" but just a fact. True balance and harmony has no 'rub', does not seek to compartmentalise and label people, situations or aspirations.

Brian, a patient I saw many years ago, was a good teacher for me. He came to me with high hopes and the work we did together helped me realise what this job is really about.

"Apparently I am firing blanks," he said with an embarrassed smile. Looking down to his knee Brian quickly changed the subject to his skiing injury.

Brian was originally sent to me by his wife when their fertility consultant had advised them that no further help was available. The cause of his infertility was unknown.

He was determined to father his own child. The impact of his infertility diagnosis was devastating to him. He felt emasculated and talked a great deal about his shame and damaged pride throughout the two years of his treatment with me. His wife was extremely supportive and understanding of how Brian felt in this situation, but was very keen to move forward with assisted fertility treatment because of her age.

After six months of acupuncture treatment Brian's

sperm sample had improved and although still far from adequate, there was enough for them to attempt ICSI. Sadly, three attempts were unsuccessful. After the final failed attempt, donor sperm was suggested as an alternative. For Brian the thought of his wife carrying another man's child was unacceptable and incredibly painful for him. He went through the emotions of someone whose partner was considering adultery, which only seemed to deepen his sense of isolation and anger.

At this stage we both agreed that our sessions were more about the emotional process of him accepting the possibility of raising a child that was not genetically his own, than about improving his fertility. This was a long and very painful process for Brian. Having never before examined or talked to anyone about his internal emotional landscape, he developed an understanding and vocabulary about himself which I doubt he would ever have imagined possible. The issues were not just about becoming a father but touched on his whole worldview: his sense of himself, his family, his relationships and career.

For Brian, agreeing to donor sperm meant giving something up. It became clear as we worked through the issues, that on some level he felt he would lose something by giving his wife the opportunity to give birth. Adoption had been considered but, like Brian, his wife wanted the experience of having her own child and did not see adoption as a favorable option. Brian had difficulty around 'give and take' in his life: a generous, open, sympathetic person by nature, he was often trapped by his own fear of missing out or not getting what he felt he needed. Through treatment I was able to help Brian develop his understanding of his and others' needs and nourishment. He was eventually able to make the great sacrifice of allowing his wife to give birth to her own child and to be there to support her as the father of their baby. Their first attempt at In-Vitro Fertilisation (IVF) using donor sperm was successful and Brian and his wife now have a beautiful son.

When I look at the work I do I can see that the outcome that is initially expected is often far from the end result of treatment, but the sessions have nevertheless been successful. In Brian's case, I believe that the difficulties which he and his wife surmounted have served to strengthen their relationship, helped develop him emotionally in a way many would never attempt, and ultimately ended with the birth of a baby.

The decision to have a baby which is not biologically your own is of course a difficult one for a woman to make too. I've talked about the culture we live in and its stress on the role of women as mothers, and many women are attacked for being "unnatural" if they don't want to have children. Worse still, some women are criticised for using medical methods or choosing an egg donor. There are all kinds of families, and all kinds of ways of conceiving children. Unless your intention is to rain terror on the world by birthing the Anti-Christ, I don't think it's up to anyone to judge what you choose to do.

There are of course those clients who do leave disappointed, upset, even angry – they had high hopes.

Often it just doesn't happen, for all the changes made. Grief follows - a clear sense of the child who was going to arrive in your life and now never will. Jennifer said, "I was absolutely furious when we stopped trying, but as time goes on ultimately I realised I have done everything I could. I've accepted it now."

For any of you who have not experienced this kind of loss, it is hard to describe the depth of pain and devastation I have witnessed some people feel. It is a strange and isolating bereavement as nothing tangible has been lost other than a thought, a hope, a dream and possibly an expectation. One of the great coping strategies for most people is to move out of grief and victimhood by recognising this truth – it was just a thought. Jennifer also coped; "If you're not given the gift of a child it doesn't mean you're not deserving, or that someone else who was given one is more deserving than you. It's just the way life is. There's no big force maliciously excluding you."

First person: Andrea

"My husband and I wanted to start having children when we got engaged, but decided to hold off until we were married. Quite soon after our wedding I was diagnosed with an auto-immune disorder called Graves Disease and had to take a course of medication that ruled out trying for a baby in the meantime, as it would have been dangerous for both me and the foetus. I'd been going back and forth to my GP with symptoms for a long time, and it was frustrating how long it took to diagnose the very classic symptoms I had. He kept

saying I must have a virus, or early on-set rheumatism.
After I finished these drugs I had radiation therapy,
which of course meant I had to delay trying for a baby
once more.

Eventually I was moved to a prescription drug that
allowed me to conceive and be pregnant without the
baby or I coming to harm, but nothing happened, so of
course we found ourselves in the long, tedious process
of doing the rounds of more doctors and more tests.
Finally they said, "We don't know what's wrong, but
you'll probably need IVF and there's a year's waiting
list." Mercifully, we were able to go privately, and start
the IVF process earlier.

I hated IVF. The first cycle felt like a last resort, like
the worst cases scenario. It was where you went when
you couldn't conceive naturally. That was just how I
saw it and I was very nervous about the whole process;
it was daunting and I didn't know what was involved.
I'd sit in the waiting room and look at all the other
women and think, "I don't want to be here, I don't want
to be another woman in an IVF clinic."

I had no sense of sisterhood or solidarity. I was
contemptuous towards them because they were infertile
women and they were my peers and I didn't want to be
one of them. I thought it was just something I'd go
through and then I'd have a child and it would all be
behind me, but this rage and anger was amplified by
the fact that all my friends were getting pregnant,
taking maternity leave and pushing babies around in
prams. As each person one by one announced their

pregnancy I could just see that statistically I was going to be the one who didn't have a kid.

It was a really dark time for me, and I did start seeing a psychotherapist, although I'm not sure quite what I got out of it other than that it took the pressure off my husband and saved my marriage. My husband was unhappy because I was depressed, and I was just leaning on him, and the best thing about the shrink was that it got me to take all that sadness out of the house and have somebody else to talk to so he didn't have to prop me up all the time. I probably got more self-knowledge and tools but I stopped going after a few years because I saw that I could be going to see her forever and ever! She was trying to get me to accept the fact that I might never have biological children, but that was just inconceivable to me. It was inconceivable that they should be inconceivable!

I started having acupuncture appointments with Gerad at this time and went five or six times, but in the end I gave up because I was just overwhelmed by everything I was going through, and the acupuncture just felt like another thing that was reminding me that I wasn't getting pregnant. I couldn't see it as part of the solution. I was already pissed off that I had to have even more treatment after all I'd been through with Graves Disease. It just seemed like more needles being stuck into me; part of the problem, rather than a solution. I was very angry with the world about everything.

All that people were saying was, "We don't know what's wrong with you, but why don't you just try relaxing because that will help." It was just such a glib thing to say, and it felt like a slap to me, as though they were saying it was my fault. "You're not getting pregnant because you're an uptight bitch!". I probably was an uptight bitch at the time!

We went through six cycles of IVF in four years, five with fresh and one with a frozen embryo. I started having treatment with Gerad again later, and it helped to calm me down and reduce the old stomach-churning anxiety. It's a cliché but after a session I'd feel like something had lifted. I don't know if it was the needles or the calm atmosphere at the clinic or the fact that I took it far more seriously than the therapy sessions, but it alleviated that very physical anxiety I'd felt.

Despite that, none of the implantations have worked out. I thought that IVF was one of those things you did and you were pregnant in no time, because I didn't know anyone who'd gone through it. Now I understand what a gamble it is, personally and financially each time you do it, and we're just about ready to give up. I know it's hard for my husband because he couldn't really do anything, and he would just have to watch this big bag of drugs arrive for me and me subjecting myself to the whole procedure and it's horrible when it doesn't work. Now we're looking seriously at adopting, and I haven't had any further goes at IVF for eight months.

It's really hard to give up though. I'm 39, and I wonder, if it worked this time, I'd have a baby in just nine months. It's not even about having our own biological children, it's just about the amount of days till we can hold our child and have a family. When you've already been waiting for years, through all these delays, it's incredibly hard to give up. Adoption will take at least two years, and it just feels like once more we're back at the drawing board, at the beginning of yet another process with new things to fathom and understand, but my friends who have adopted are right: at least you know there's a child at the end of it, unlike IVF.

The last time we went to a fertility clinic to hear the results of tests to work out why the IVF had failed, we were almost excited because we thought that finally a doctor would tell us that they'd found the problem and we definitely couldn't have biological children, and then we would go on and adopt without a backward glance. In the end they said what they always said; that we were healthy, my eggs had a full set of chromosomes, and that we should try again. It actually felt like bad news.

When we've marked a year without medical fertility treatment we can begin the process of adoption. The acupuncture and chat I've had with Gerad since that last trip to the IVF clinic has been all about balancing me out and thinking about what life will be like without my own birth children, and just concentrating on making me a happier and less stressed person above all. I'm going to need to make some changes to my life, like perhaps finding a new career, because though I love my job it stresses me out. The important thing is to know that we have lots of options and that everything is open. I've now realised that not having a kid is not the only reason why I'm unhappy and anxious so much of the time. I can't rely on getting pregnant to make myself a happy person. I have to take responsibility for being happier. There's more to life than having biological children, and you can't control everything in your world. It's taken a long time for me to get to a place where I can accept that I won't carry and give birth to my own children; it was just too painful to imagine for a long time, and it was something that I'd assumed always, always, always, would happen for us. We don't want to go into adoption thinking it's the second best thing, just with some trepidation. I do feel quite confident and positive about it in a way that I didn't feel a year ago. I don't think "Oh poor me, what more do I have to go through?". I think, "Blimey, this is going to be hectic but really exciting." It's finally something positive, and when I hear stories about people who have adopted kids, I just think it's amazing and so lovely.

Now there's a part of me that can go down that hippy route and think, maybe we weren't supposed to have our own children because there are some children out there who need us like we need them. Matt and I need a family, and those children need a family, and we just need to come together."

First person: Jack *"My fertility didn't change. At a certain point I thought "Acupuncture isn't working for my fertility, but it's certainly working for the rest of my life". I wasn't upset that I didn't have a cure, but I was glad I got something out of it for my general well being.*

229

One positive outcome of my infertility was that it forced my wife and I to tackle issues in our relationship that we hadn't quite dealt with up till then. It made us sit down and re-evaluate what we wanted and how we worked together. We needed to be really close and really aligned, really connected to proceed in having kids in a way that was going to be much more difficult and challenging than we'd expected.

There's this whole guy thing about passing on your name, and fortunately it was never that important to me, but I understand if you feel like something's dying out with you, but to be honest, once you have your kids and they're walking around and talking and doing things with you, I don't think it matters very much.

Our eldest child is a donor insemination baby, and my wife carried him and gave birth to him. After he was born she got pregnant in the same way with sperm from the same donor, but miscarried, after which we learned that she would be unable to have any more children. It was an incredibly difficult time, to take a second major diagnosis like this, but I think the fact that we'd been through it before with me helped. It seemed easier to move on to adoption for our second child.

It took two years at least, and just when we'd given up on it ever happening, we were told there was a three-month-old baby for us to adopt. Adoption is difficult and it's hit and miss with a lot of uncertainty because they're not sure if they'll have a kid for you and then, suddenly, boom! Three weeks later you take him home! It's crazy! It's crazy emotionally and practically but that's what it is, and it's amazing.

We got a real mixed bag, but we also got the family that was in our vision. It took a lot of grief and pain and sadness, but it doesn't really matter how you get them once they're running around your house.

People think if they have a birth child they'll know what they'll get, but they won't! There are a lot of issues physical or mental that a kid can have, whether you adopt them or conceive them naturally. Having kids is a crapshoot, and will ever be thus! Children are not really yours anyway. They're their own people and they're going to run off eventually – you just have them for a while. It's what all biological parents end up having to learn, but when you have an adopted child, you know it from the start and can give them space to be themselves."

Sometimes our options are restricted by a set of circumstances beyond our control, like, for example, an intractable physical problem that makes conception impossible, as it was for Jack. When this happens we have to make allowances and work within those restrictions, but we should always avoid making false restrictions for ourselves. Life does not have to be "just so" as we wanted it to be. Life requires us to be flexible, and sometimes we have to change our goals and what we're reaching for too.

First person: Martin *"My wife and I knew quite early on that we didn't want to go through IVF, and that we weren't desperate and would be happy to be just the two of us, and we still had a lot to live for. We turned to adoption, and to an excellent voluntary*

231

agency. We had a lot of friends who had adopted as role models, and didn't feel that we had to pass on our genes to a biological child in order to be parents.

The process took about two years, and we had to swear off having any further fertility treatment. You have to resolve the whole notion of having biological kids for yourself, which I know can be very hard for men and women. I wouldn't say we're grieving now for a birth child we never had, but at some point in the process you do have to come to terms with the fact that you're putting that idea behind you.

The agency we signed up with put us through a home study that asked us to look deep within ourselves and be absolutely honest about what we could cope with as parents. No child these days comes without a certain amount of baggage, and you feel you ought to be able to be a parent to anybody, but you're not doing anyone any favours by taking that attitude, because if you're not honest about what you can deal with, you'll let the child down.

Between the treatment with Gerad and the adoption process, I took stock of my life, and I've definitely changed. When it began I was working for an organisation that consumed a lot of my physical and emotional energy, and now I'm self-employed and very engaged in the upbringing of my son. I practice mindfulness to keep myself on track.

Not having a birth child becomes irrelevant as soon as you have your adopted child: there's the child and it needs you and you just form an attachment. My son was four months old when we first met him with his foster *carers, and there was just an instant bond that felt physical. He fell asleep on my shoulder, and it was incredible that he felt comfortable enough to do that."*

One couple came to see me soon after they married. They had met relatively late in their lives, and knew it was unlikely that they would be able to have children, but thought they would try anyway. They were such rational, loving people, and because they barely seemed to need my help as they had accepted the fact that they might not have kids and it didn't bother them. They were so happy to be together that they knew they would have a nice life regardless.

After a few months they arrived at the clinic one day and told me that they'd decided not to adopt children, but to offer themselves as foster parents instead. I asked why, and they said that as they were both older they thought it was just something they would be able to offer, especially to teenage children. Once they had made up their minds they moved very quickly and smoothly through the processes required by social services, and although they no longer came for treatment, they stayed in touch to let me know how much they were enjoying their new role giving a secure home to sometimes very challenging adolescents.

Kate was a big hitter in a government department when she met her partner, Bruno in her late twenties, and they'd been happily together for several years before she arrived at the clinic looking for help with having a baby. She was very dynamic, and very ambitious at work, and one of the things she told me in the first consultation was that she had never considered having children, but now she'd been made to realise that she had to think about it now, or else miss an opportunity. There was a sudden wave of pressure from family and friends wanting to know when they'd have children, with the general consensus being that no job and no marriage could be so enthralling that it would be as satisfying as having kids. They were both from big families. She'd been told that once she had a baby in her arms she'd feel differently. She'd spoken with Bruno and they'd decided to go for it, but you couldn't mistake their ambivalence. They had developed a certain determination though, although it felt like a box ticking exercise, a challenge that they had taken on for the sake of it. She rallied and got fully behind it, but it wasn't happening.

I thought she was great. She was one of those genuinely strong people who are well in their own skin; she was not suffering from any kind of spiritual crisis. There was nothing really wrong with her and she wasn't in denial about anything, except perhaps this ambivalent attitude to conceiving. Kate wasn't interested in the idea that maybe it wouldn't happen if she didn't want it deep down, and now that it was becoming a challenge, she wanted to overcome it as she'd done problems at work. "I'll just get on with it and see what happens," she told me.

After two years, the baby project was heading towards "failure". Bruno had become so caught up in the process that he was making charts and timing their sex life, and their previously close-knit relationship was showing the strain. The whole thing had started to be very uncomfortable, and I felt as though I was treating her just in an effort to stop her falling into this self-created problem. They'd set themselves up for failure in something that had never really cared about much in the first place. I questioned my own ability to treat her because I was treating something that wasn't there. I just wanted to keep her as strong as she was when she first arrived for a consultation.

Suddenly she disappeared for a few months and I wondered what had happened. One minute she wasn't there and the next she was back at the clinic, telling me that she had quit her job. She and Bruno were going to move back to his home country of Italy and set up a nursery for local children. They'd started using contraception again and didn't want to have children.

Why on earth did she want to work with kids then, I asked, and she said she just wanted a business and she loved being around kids, even if she was happy to go home without them at the end of the day. What had first seemed bizarre was actually a perfect ending: it was clean, satisfactory and sorted. It was a huge life change, but they've been now there for 5 years and are thriving. I sometimes wonder what would have happened if she had conceived, but in the end just the idea of a baby was enough to open the possibility for an incredible life change and fresh challenges.

The Gift

We live in a world of good and bad, light and shade, war and peace; a world of duality where nothing is static and which exists only by the virtue of this ever present tension. Nature is this reaction; a constantly shifting, vibrant, energised life force tipping and turning as it seeks the centre ground, the point of balance, our true self. What we witness in nature is a sophisticated complex system in constant flow, moving between chaos and order but always returning to a state of balance.

The human spirit is part of the same force that makes all life possible and which directs nature and the natural world around us, bringing back to that easy equilibrium. I've tried to explain how, in Taoist philosophy, we are part of nature, born of it, maintained by it and subject to its laws, and that trusting our spirit's guidance and strength is fundamental to us. We need to be in a relationship with spirit and work from this place, so that rather than strive in the world to find peace, we start from peace as we strive.

We all have the capacity to be healthy, content and productive human beings. Even after years of depression or health problems we still have that positive potential. A seed can lie dormant for years waiting for the conditions to be right and then it has the energy to sprout.

You can choose from a great array of practitioners and books and services to help you in the process, but none of us can fix you, ultimately. I don't believe that fertility gurus exist. There are people who are prepared to serve and help people and there are people who share wisdom. They are ordinary people who give good advice. They can help you discover a way forward, and a way to negotiate emotional and physical changes, but without your own efforts to listen to yourself, their help will go nowhere. They will not and cannot fix you. That is your responsibility, although they can help when that responsibility feels too much to bear.

Our role is to give you a sense of perspective if you need it, to stand back and take a good, subjective look at your life, your thoughts and feelings and to see what drives them. Is your true underlying instinct or sense of self there, or are you pursuing/battling for something that you don't want deep down? It's a cliché to say "be yourself" but one that's barely understood in its true meaning. All I can do as a practitioner is to try to help to bring balance and harmony and hopefully witness the truth revealed. An element imbalance in wood, fire, earth, metal or water is only one way for that knot to manifest itself.

I do believe that we all have the ability to change, but change is often difficult. By the time we have left our childhood, struggled through puberty and found our way in the world, we have created our own personal reality. Our friendships, sexual relationships, career paths, personal ideologies and morality form the foundation of the personal perspective that frames our life experience. What we perceive through these windows appears to be real and fixed. For some of us the view is pleasant and easy, for others it is difficult and troubled but it is our view and of our making based

237

on our reactions to the outside world. Faced with a traumatic event in our lives, we have a choice in how we react and what we do with this experience. This event could be used to back up an already crystallised view that life is painful and difficult. Conversely the experience could be seen as an opportunity to learn and change our core beliefs and perspective. Without making a judgement of the right or wrong way it does suggest we have choice and that our choices will affect our future.

There is the story of the victim who gets to blame something or someone else, and the story of the brave survivor who battles on in the face of childlessness and is just "fine". These stories come from the negative part of us which is invested in pain and suffering, one which converts pain into a kind of pride and face saving exercise. These stories do nothing to help us reach fulfilment because they trap us in either a passive role (the specialists will do it all) or define us by a single failure. The third story is that of the person who knows their self and the truth, and draws on their own resources to roll with the punches or to appreciate the good times when they come. When you can be yourself you are empowered, there are no obstacles to your natural inclinations, your personality - your spirit.

It really comes down to how much personal responsibility you are prepared to take, although few people understand what that really means. It doesn't mean being a captain of industry with two hundred employees under you and the buck stopping at your desk. It means owning your own feelings and thoughts, and being a person who is accountable to your self. Our best resources are found inside us, and we already have everything we need.

This book is full of stories of people who were pleasantly surprised to discover that the life they'd thought they wanted wasn't necessarily the best for them after all. They left desirable jobs, quit their nice houses, even left the country and began doing something completely different or found children who needed them to be their parents. Equally there are stories of people who stopped competing and searching and started to enjoy the life they already had. And once they all discovered their own unique truth, they settled and got underway to observe life unfold with or without children.

When confronted with something as emotive as believing that we might not be able to have our own child, an opportunity arises. We realise that we are not perfect; and what a gift that is. As Leonard Cohen says in his moving song 'Anthem'; "There is a crack in everything – that's how the light gets in".

Tools for Balance

The "tools" listed below are based on the advice I have given the countless "baby-making" people I have helped for over the past 20 years. They are tried and tested, and from the feedback I have received they appear to have been enormously beneficial in helping people reach their goal. They are all based on common sense and will not necessarily be new to you, but implementing them on a daily basis possibly will be. I strongly encourage you to give them a try.

Drinking Water

Have you ever sat by a large body of water and listened to the sound? Even with gentle rolling waves it can sound like four jumbo jets flying overhead. Next time you are at the beach, listen. Not only will you hear the relentless and powerful sound of waves dragging the sand backwards and forwards, but an echo of greatness that fills the entire space. The immense power of oceans and rivers can be totally overwhelming, as we have seen in recent years with the tsunamis that have devastated human life in a matter of minutes, and yet we see this awe inspiring power and force of nature as something outside of ourselves.

We are primarily made of space, but after that, the majority of our physical form is water - something around 75% of our body mass - and this is the same water you see in the sea, the rain, the snow and the sweat on your forehead recycled and shared amongst every living thing in the earth's atmosphere. We are powerful beings! It's astonishing to realise that the water you drank this morning (if you did of course) is the same water that dinosaurs were quenching their thirst on millions of years ago.

Water is the origin of life as we know it. We are born of water, grow from water and are sustained throughout our lives by water. All of the attributes of water we witness in nature are present in us – droughts creating dry skin and constipation, fast flowing rivers delivering hormones and flushing in new ideas, tsunamis producing searing headaches and panic attacks, mountain top lakes bringing freshness – a peace of mind.

As we are all so painfully aware, as we get older we lose our ability to retain water – we dry up – and along with this natural dehydrating process that will eventually take us to our graves, we lose the vital and essential energy that created us in the first place, that powers our life and our ability to contribute to the creation of new life. The power of conception and creation, that feeds and divides every cell is rooted in this element and by no coincidence is stronger and more abundant when we are young. I can remember in my teens, 20's and early 30's never drinking any water. Why would I? I never felt thirsty and rarely felt tired. Not only that, late nights, alcohol and emotional chaos didn't seem to stop most of us from conceiving and producing beautiful bouncing babies. Oh, but we were young. As much as it might be fashionable, P.C. and comforting to shy away for the truth that conception is easier in young people, we must face reality. The good news is that from my experience of helping the chronically dehydrated over 30's with fertility problems, age is not so much of a concern but proper hydration is.

As I have explained, the nature of water is not just to moisturise, it is nature's medicine. Water lubricates, brings power, cleanses, promotes movement, strengthens, balances, dilutes, provides buoyancy…and the list goes on. It is nothing short of miraculous and yet many of my patients often complain when I offer them what I think might be the secret to all their problems and ask them to drink water – they say they are not thirsty. If I bottled it and sold it as an infertility cure I would most likely have enormous success and become a millionaire overnight. People trawl the web looking for the next best substance to ingest in their quest for premium health and optimum fertility and yet their foundation is not in place. For many of us, our body gave up asking for water many years ago after we managed to convince it there was a massive drought and to make do with what it has.

I feel so passionately about this that I will go as far to say that everything – and I mean everything, is dependent on this element. Every new treatment, every new habit, every new strategy you employ to conceive will ultimately fail unless you give yourself this foundation for life. From an acupuncture point of view it's essential. The acupuncture needles can move the formless energy in the channels, but this effect needs to filter down to the material level, and this is water. Water is the basis of blood, which in turn feeds our muscles, our tendons and ligaments, our skin, our reproductive organs – every part of us.

"My doctor told me I get enough water from food and drinks", she protested. "It just won't go down, I can't swallow it", he said having told me he drinks three pints of beer every night. "It doesn't taste of anything", she complained, "and it's too cold". "But wine and whiskey is made of water!" he said looking at me suspiciously - and so the protests and excuses go on and on. All of the above may be true but what we do know is that dehydration is life threatening and it is only a few steps back from that where we can see it as "new-life threatening". The debate continues and all the fertility experts have their own ideas about water but become your own expert and spend some time in nature and see what happens when water is abundant.

Eating Breakfast

"Breakfast like a King or Queen". Yes - it's as simple as that! We are designed by Nature to transform food into life-giving energy between the hours of 7am and 9am. Much like the list of excuses I have already described for not drinking water, a more imaginative and colourful list is conjured up when I encourage people to eat a big breakfast. It would be amusing if the people protesting were not the one's who are hoping to create new life.

I do understand that if it is something you have never done, it will feel strange at first. Your stomach deprived of its primary function for over maybe 30 years is suddenly asked to perform, and of course, it goes into shock. So start simply with bite size chunks and wean yourself gently in until you are truly feasting every morning. Remember the Law of Midday/Midnight and how by ignoring this natural law to eat at this time can disrupt every action for the remainder of your day.

Menu of the Day
- Breakfast like a King or Queen – Fats, Carbohydrates and Protein
- Lunch like a Prince or Princess – Carbohydrates and Protein
- Supper like pauper - Protein

True Rest

We're all very busy - running around, working, socialising, jumping up and down, having sex, travelling, cleaning – you name it – we're doing it. Yet, rest and downtime is often very low on our agenda of important daily activities. Understandably – there's a lot to do.

Doing nothing is often considered a "waste of time" and the idea that we could just sit in a chair and do nothing for an hour is not only verging on sinful but for some of us it's impossible. The Western work ethic is still strong in many of us despite the decline of its righteous roots, and like all habits, the habit of busyness is hard to break when our culture encourages and congratulates us for every extra hour we keep ourselves turned "on".

Providing we have a relatively good night's rest, a lie-in on a Sunday and a couple of weeks on a beach somewhere once in a while, we consider this to be enough. The truth is that most of us are deeply tired and running on empty. One of the ways I make a diagnosis when working as an acupuncturist is to read the "pulses" of the patient to establish the strength and the balance of their energy. It amazes me that people are even able to make it to my treatment room, let alone do all the things I've listed above. The problem we face is that we are not even aware of how exhausted we really are. I mentioned earlier in the book the frog in the pot that slowly gets cooked without even knowing the heat's on. The same is true here but the other way round. We get used to our low reserves and compensate with substances, adrenaline and sheer grit. The other problem is, that just like a car, the petrol gauge may be near empty but the car will keep running at full speed - until it stops. Running an efficient menstrual cycle, maturing eggs and sperm, conceiving and making a baby all take a lot of energy. Make sure "you put a tiger in your tank".

Here are my tips for getting good rest and building your reserves.

- Observe good sleep hygiene

The bedroom is for sex and sleep only. Don't hang out in there, reading, watching TV or chatting on the phone.

- Be asleep by 11pm

You will remember the Chinese Clock that teaches us the importance of getting to bed early and being asleep by 11pm. Start the natural sleep cycles on time, essential for your regeneration, which will in turn benefit all your organs and functions that follow for the rest of the 24 hour cycle.

- Get up at the same time every day

Choose a time to get up (ideally no later than 7am) and stick to it every day. There is room for some flexibility but the more routine your body is given, the better quality of sleep you will enjoy.

- Take time to sit – meditate

Sitting or meditating is a great bridge between our unconscious and conscious states. Getting up and immediately rushing around, listening to the radio, checking emails is not the best way to start the day. Sitting or meditating for 10 minutes soon after waking is a wonderful way to bring the restful and peaceful state of sleep into the waking day. Sit quietly and focus on the in-breath and the out-breath and put your attention on the stillness that exists within you and away from the busyness of your mind. Repeat this throughout the day – even 5 minutes is enough.

- Be mindful in all you do

This is an extension of a sitting - meditative practice. It simply means being fully present and more conscious of your life as it unfolds. It is easy to be distracted by thoughts and spend the whole day in your head. It's exhausting. Take each activity as it comes and be fully present to it without judgement. Brushing your teeth is just as valid as the next big deal.

- Find an activity that brings you "true rest"

"True Rest" is not necessarily about going to sleep or napping. We all have something we do that we recognise is good for us. I enjoy taking my dog for a walk, or going for a swim, and I'm aware that after these activities I feel better. It's very subjective and it is important that you decide which ones works for you. Some people find reading books brings "true rest", for others it's stressful. Whatever it is, become aware of it and integrate it into your life as a priority. The quality

of all your other activities will immediately benefit
from it.

The Pendulum

The Pendulum is a wonderful tool - simple, transformational and extremely effective.

Our thoughts and feelings are in a constant state of flux – impermanent, changeable, sometimes volatile and often unpredictable. They can swing from one polarity to the next, from good to bad, from right to wrong, happy to sad and somewhere in-between. The pendulum represents our thoughts and feelings in flux. Imagine a pendulum; the fine end hangs from a fixed point, its heavy counterpoint moving as it swings from one polarity to the next, but ultimately always settling at the midpoint – the calm. In good health, when a happy event occurs, or you have a joyful thought, your pendulum swings towards the "good", and once acknowledged you naturally gravitate back to home base - the calm. Maybe a friend loses a parent, or perhaps you fall and hurt your self - the pendulum heads to the "bad", but once again, when in good health, once felt, you head back to the calm. And so it goes on, constantly moving from one appropriate response to the next.

The reality, however, for most of us is very different, we get stuck or become attached to one side of the pendulum or the other – we have preferences, more often than not favouring the good, but also, at times, favouring the bad. The "compulsive swingers", of course, love the ride so much they swing madly from one side to the next, rarely visiting the midpoint or the calm at all.

The purpose of the pendulum as a "tool" is for us to use it to develop an awareness of how our thoughts and feelings can take over and control our life. We generally tend to keep the swing to one side or the other because we believe that we are caught in a world that only offers us an either/or option. The pendulum teaches us we can have both.

By climbing up the pendulum like a monkey scales a tree, on reaching the top, we realise we can think or feel good or bad - and still experience the calm. We spend our lives clinging to the base of the pendulum cooking up strategies to keep us in one place or another when it really doesn't matter when you're viewing it from the top.

The golden rule of the pendulum is that you should never make a decision or take action at either end of the swing. By all means enjoy the experience of each extreme, but always bring it back home to the calm before you take your next step.

A Note about J R Worsley

Jack Reginald Worsley, known as J.R, is the man credited with bringing Five-Element acupuncture to the Western World. The son of an engineer with an interest in Chinese philosophy, he first worked in a factory before being enlisting as an Army Education Officer in the British Army during the Second World War. He later became a physiotherapist and an osteopath and began to investigate alternative medical practices including acupuncture, but it was not until he travelled in Singapore, Taiwan and Korea in the 1950s that he discovered the Five-Element style of acupuncture. He studied and became a "master" and on his return to the UK, founded a school to pass on the teachings he had learned.

In 1986 I was treated for the first time by a Five-Element practitioner in San Francisco, where I was living at that time. I sought treatment because I was feeling very unwell and had just been given a medical diagnosis that suggested my life span could be severely compromised. The day after my first treatment I remember feeling profoundly different. I was somewhat perplexed by the striking result of what seemed like just a few random needles but I was excited, intrigued and keen to discover more. My practitioner at the time had been trained by Professor Worsley himself, who suggested I return to the UK to study at Worsley's college in Leamington Spa. By the time I enrolled Worsley had already trained hundreds of practitioners now working worldwide.

The man was brilliant. He stood miles apart from all

other teachers at his college and taught this system of medicine in such a simple way, he used to say a child of five would understand him better than any of us as we struggled to accept the discipline of simplicity. Keeping things simple, experiencing life as it is, is a skill we seem to lose as we develop our own understanding of our world. My training became an exercise in reawakening my senses and experiencing my world and the people around me with the same awe and wonder I had as a child.

J R Worsley died in 2003 and is survived by his wife Judy Becker Worsley, now the recognised leader of the Worsley Five-Element tradition. Just prior to Professor Worsley's death the Worsley Institute was formed in the U.S as a not-for-profit organisation to preserve and showcase Worsley's heritage.

www.worsleyinstitute.com.